Copyright Notice

Disclaimer Notice

Special Thanks:
Drs. Wendell Wall and
Denise McSherry

Use the Other Half of Your Brain!

About the Author and the Book

Welcome to the illustrated study guide to the Obstetrics and Gynecology Boards!

There are many theories on ways of learning and many come and go as quickly as fashion fads. However, one that persists is related to learning through visualization. This theory was introduced by Allan Pavio and is known as the "Dual Coding Theory" of learning. The idea, greatly simplified, is when we employ multiple parts of our brain to learn something, or code the information in more than one way, it is more likely to be recalled. Our working memory, or what we use when we are learning something in the "now", only holds on to a limited amount of information, such as what is needed to carry out an immediate task. However, our brains are always recording other information such as place, time, temperature and other variables. If we recognize these other informational tags and tie them to what we are learning in the now, we can better retain the memory. By using visualization and other cues we can lock-in more recall and embed the memory in different ways.

The next step would be to apply creativity or imagination to learning and this uses a different type of memory storage. Dr. Tesler used his imagination to create the imagery within this book. We would encourage you to visualize these images as you learn the topic and truly lock-in the topics being covered.

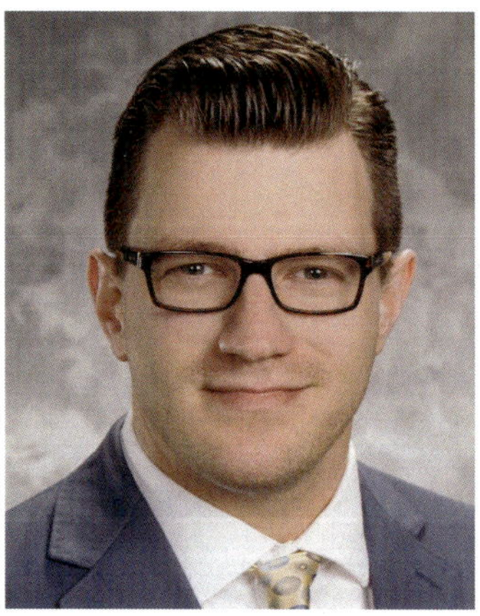

Dr. Tesler a graduate of Michigan State University, College of Human Medicine and is now a faculty physician at Central Michigan University in Obstetrics and Gynecology. He has always been interested in different modes of learning and how residents and medical students can maximize their time learning.

He began doodling to help with his own learning and often joked, "I learn best like a kindergartner!" Meaning the colors and pictures locked-in his memories the best.

He began using more drawings in his lectures while training as a resident and later when training residents as faculty. He noticed, the residents remained more engaged, enjoyed learning and increased retention of the material.

Enjoy!

OBSTETRICS

Fetal Circulation

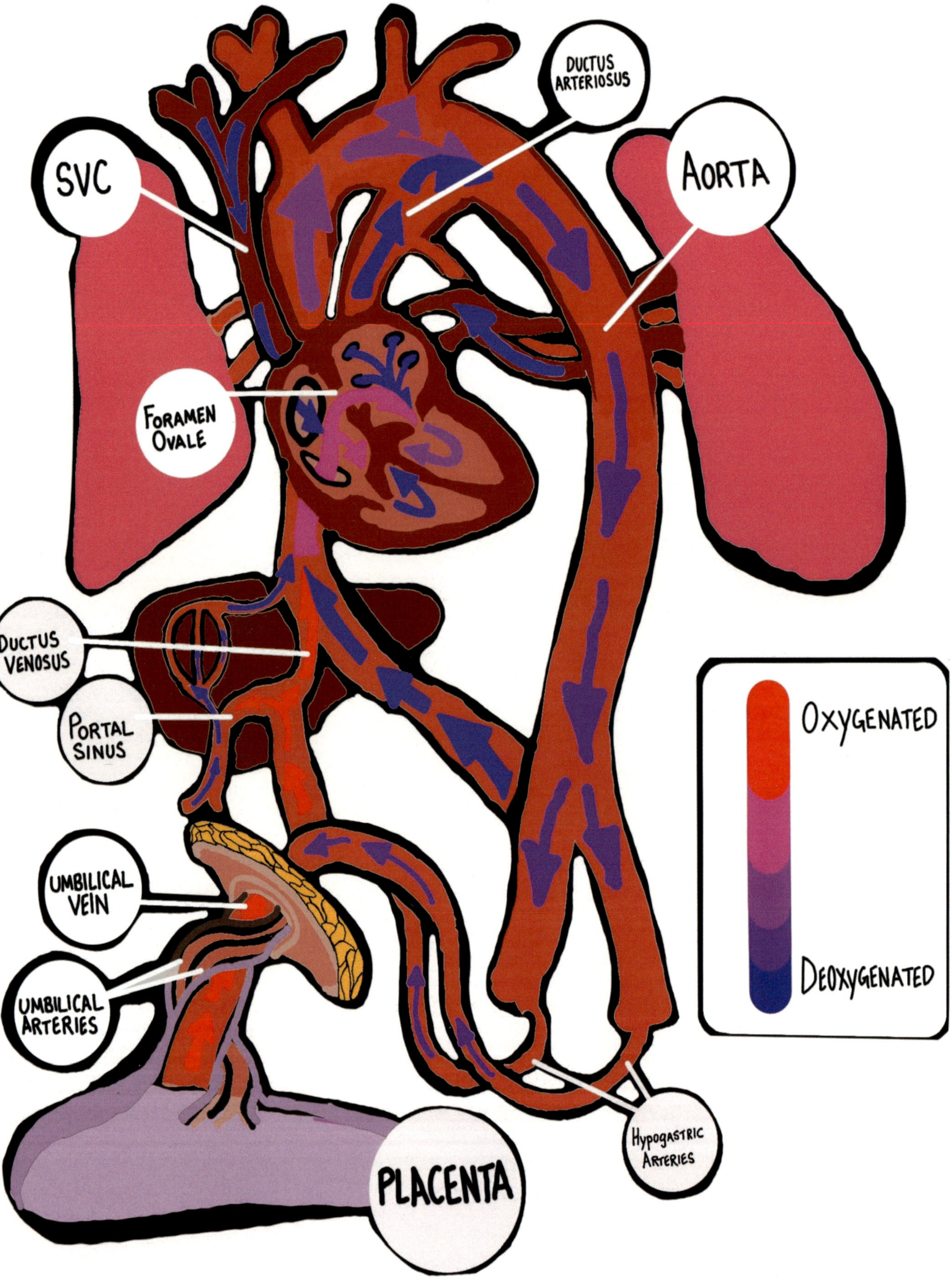

Fetal Heart and Fetal Oxygenation During Pregnancy

The fetal heart during pregnancy has many unique adaptations that allow for oxygenation throughout the pregnancy via the flow through the umbilical cord. After birth, oxygenation is occurring in the fetal lung and nutrient absorption is taking place via the gastrointestinal tract.

The Main Adaptations of Change in Fetal Circulation are:

1. The Foramen Ovale (FO) - between the Right and Left Atrium
2. The Ductus Arteriosus (DA) - between the Pulmonary Arteries and the Aorta
3. The Ductus Venosus (DV) - communication within the liver between the Inferior Vena Cava (IVC) and Portal System
4. The Umbilical Cord (Inclusive of 1 Vein and 2 Arteries)

The placental interface is a complex interchange between the fetal blood and that of its mother. After the placental exchange occurs, the blood enters the umbilical vein (which, there is 1) and proceeds towards the fetus via the umbilical cord. After entry through the umbilicus the fetal blood becomes highly oxygenated through the umbilical vein to the fetal liver.

Here the majority of this highly oxygenated and nutrient rich blood bypasses the liver via the Ductus Venosus (DV) to the Inferior Vena Cava (IVC). Remember the blood has already been loaded with nutrients from the placental interface and does not require time in the hepatic system.

The blood from the DV now intermixes with deoxygenated blood from the fetal circulation and the blood becomes partially oxygenated.

The Inferior Vena Cava carries the blood to the Right Atrium, however the blood is oxygenated and does not require the journey through the heart and pulmonary system. Thus it is shunted to the Left Atrium via the Foramen Ovale (FO). This blood is then sent through the Left Ventricle and is pumped into the fetal Aorta. Some of the blood does travel through the Right Atrium and Ventricle to the pulmonary circulation. It collects some CO_2, however, no oxygenation takes place. The Ductus Arteriosus (DA) further allows partially oxygenated blood that entered the right tract of the heart and the pulmonary circulation to bypass the lungs and enter the fetal circulation via the Aorta.

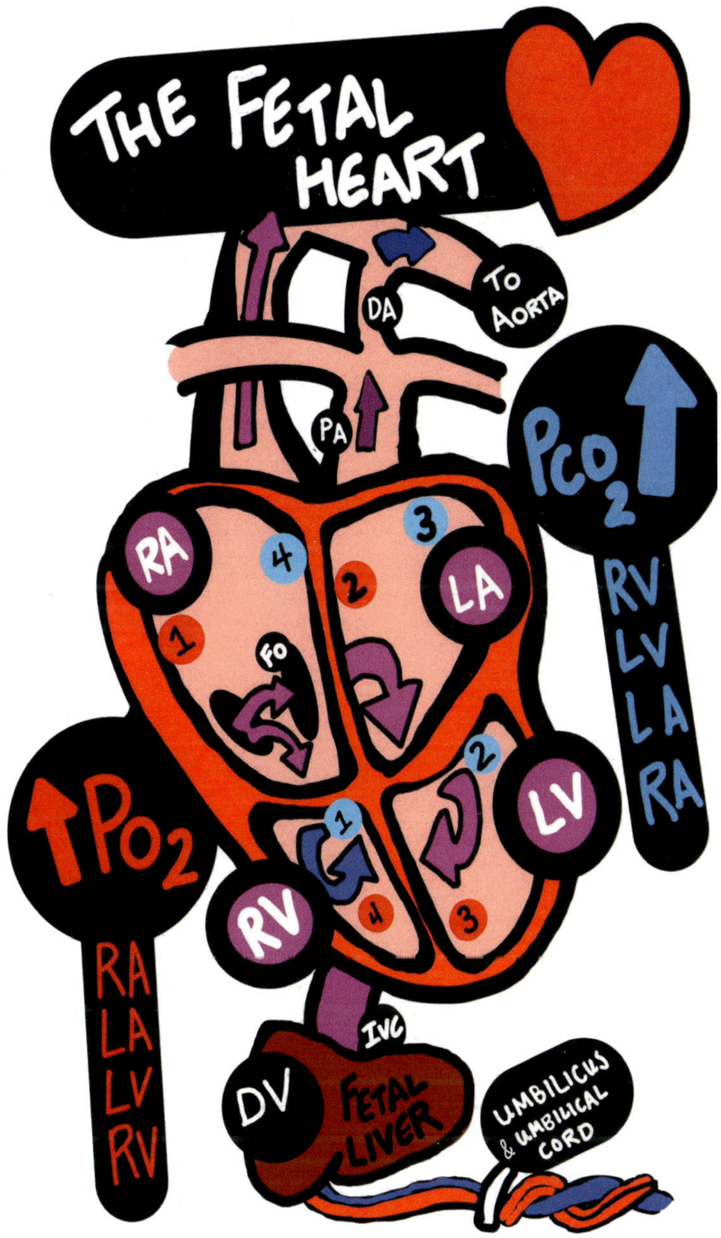

Fetal Placenta and Crossing Mechanisms

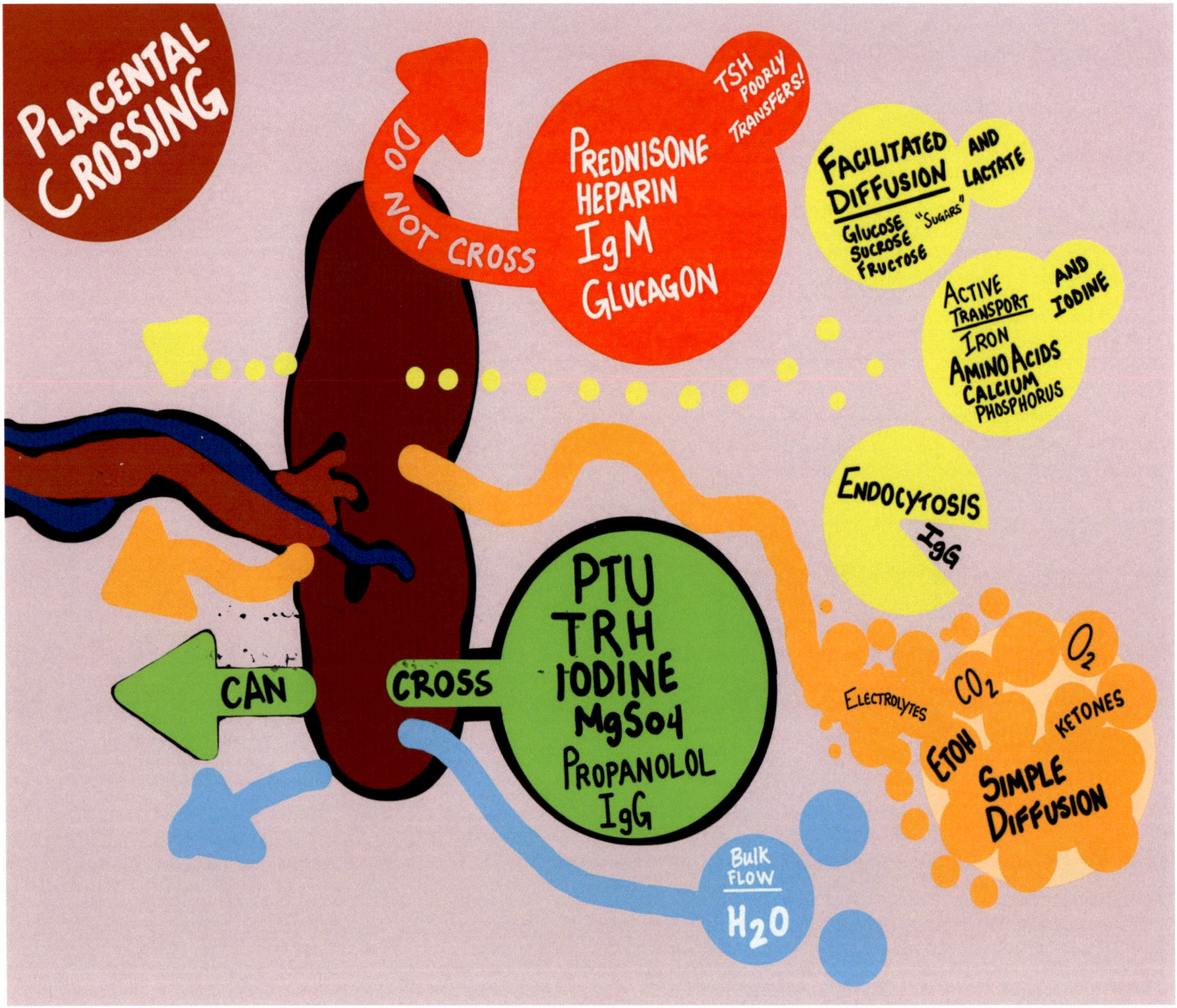

The placenta is a unique and amazing part of pregnancy physiology. It is imperative to understand what substances can cross and those that cannot. Large molecules, for example IgM, cannot cross the placental barrier to the fetal circulation, whereas IgG can GO (G) freely across the placenta.

Pay special attention to those medications that can and cannot cross the placenta as board questions will focus on these type of substances.

The placenta also produces hormones. Including: Human Chorionic Gonadotropin (hCG), Placental Lactogen (PL), Adrenocorticotropin Hormone (ACTH), Corticotropin Releasing Hormone (CRH), Gonadotropin Releasing Hormone (GnRH), Thyrotropin (TRH), Growth Hormone Releasing Hormone (GHRH), Growth Hormone Variant (hGH-V), Neuropeptide Y, Parathyroid Releasing Hormone (PTRH), Activin and Inhibin. Know these hormones!

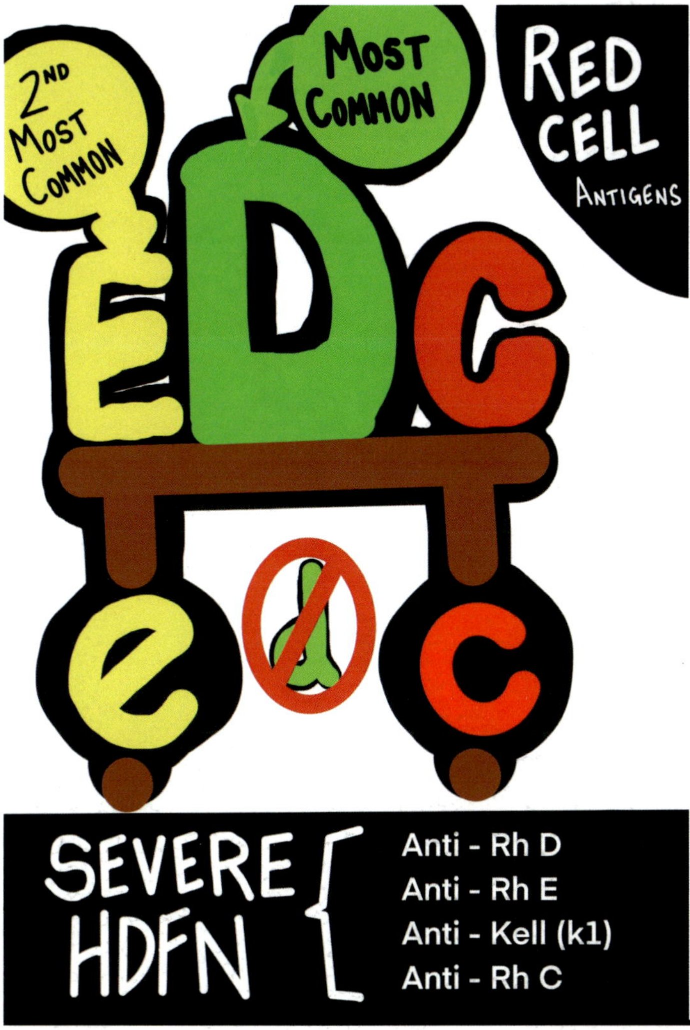
2ND MOST COMMON
MOST COMMON
RED CELL ANTIGENS
E
D
C
e
d
c
SEVERE HDFN
Anti - Rh D
Anti - Rh E
Anti - Kell (k1)
Anti - Rh C

Hemolytic Disease of the Fetus and Newborn (HDFN)

Understanding the Rh system and the Hemolytic Diseases that arise in pregnancy is important as these can quickly have extremely poor outcomes including death.

"D" is the most common red cell antigen identified in pregnancy. Notice the table has two legs, the little "e" and little "c" antigens. However, the little "d" is crossed out because there isn't one.

The most severe forms of HDFN are as listed in the bottom of the drawing. Often these diseases/antigens are monitored by titers (titration labs). The more the antigen takes to "titrate it out" of the solution, the more concerning. Thus, a 1:4 is less concerning than a 1:8. Most labs use 1:16 as the cut-off for a critical level. Some of the more severe antigens such as Anti-Kell, are usually a lower value.

ABO incompatibility is MCC of HDN (newborn)?
1:8 = critical titer of Kell ab.
1:32 = critical titer for other abs

Risk of Aneuploidy

As a woman ages the chance of a pregnancy with an aneuploidy increases. Down's Syndrome risk is a common clinical question and is frequently seen on the board exams.

Remember - the ages in the image: 30, 35 ,40 , 45

Remember - the numbers of the Down's denominators: 1,000, 365, 100, 36

All you have to do to know any other risk outside of Down's is to cut the Down's Denominators in half.

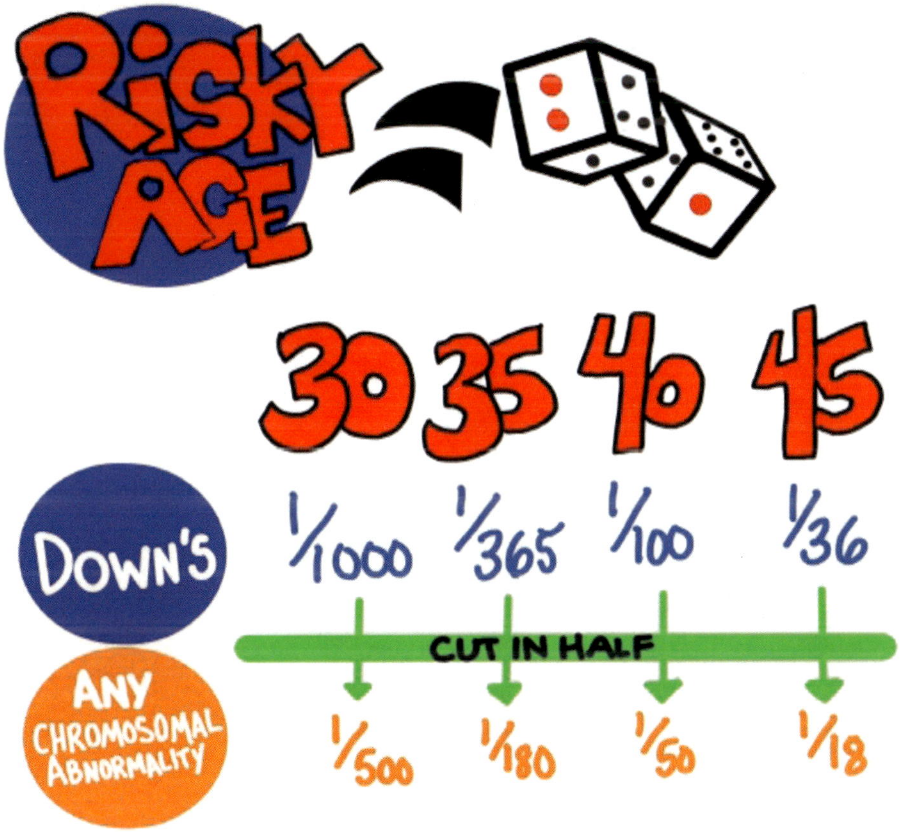

Twins and Multiples

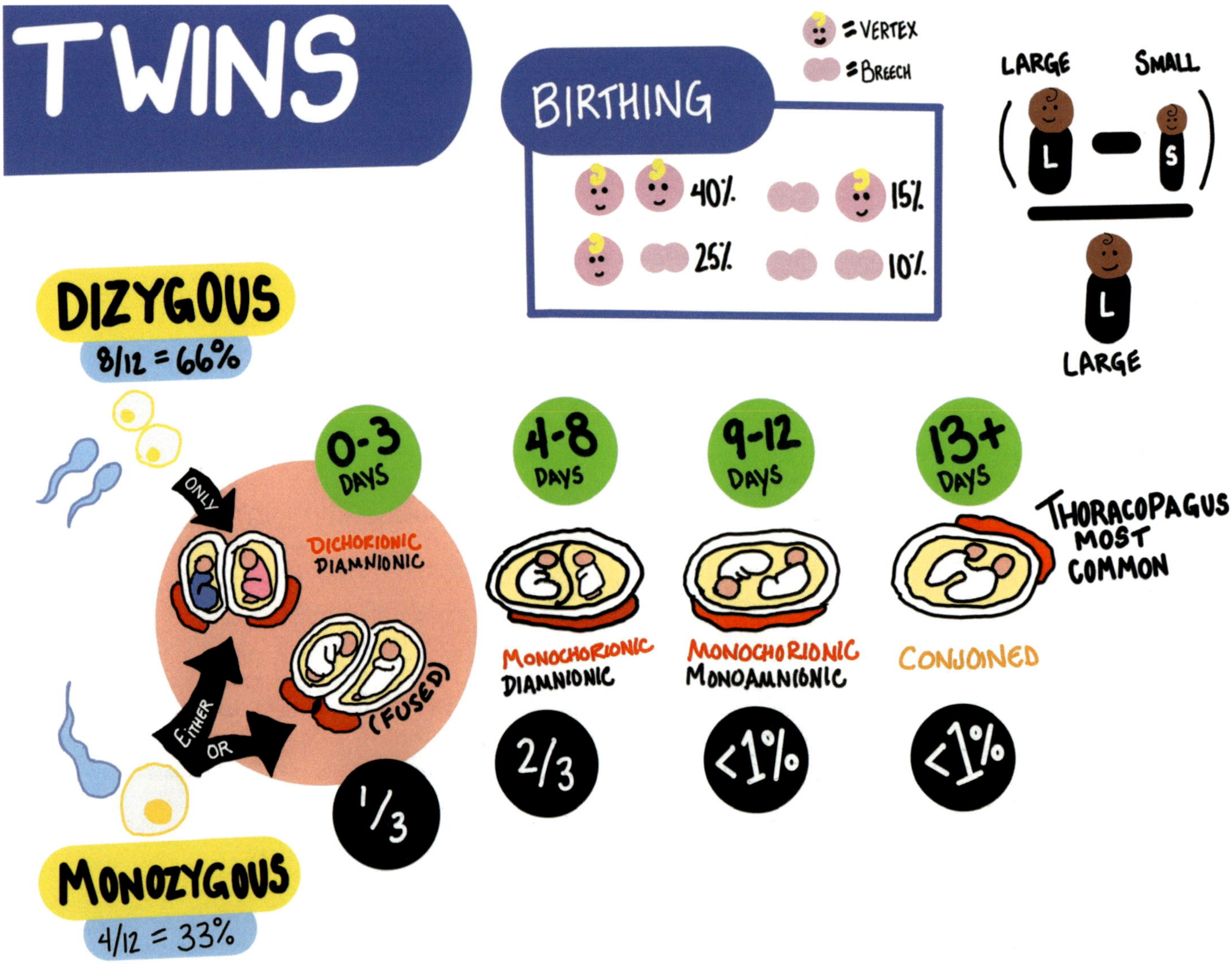

With all the inherent risks that come with multiples pregnancy, whether naturally achieved, via In Vitro Fertilization, or by medications, they are always found on the exams. Per the CDC, the current birth rate of twins in the United States is approximately 12 in 1,000 births. For triplets and higher, the birth rate is approximately 101.4 in 100,000 live births (or significantly less than twins).

Twin pregnancies have their zygosity determined by the amount of gametes that participate in the creation of the twins. Monozygotic pregnancies are created by two fetuses resulting from the fertilization of one sperm and one egg. The easiest way to determine zygosity is whether the fetuses are of a different sex, which would make them dizygotic. We know this because if there is one of each sex, there had to be two sperms that contributed an X and Y each. This could not occur in a monozygotic pregnancy.

The amount of days the division occurs from fertilization determines the chorionicity and amnionicity of the twin pregnancy.

Here is a little mnemonic to help you remember:
"By 3 we dance in our own little corners (Di/Di), by 8 we can come just a little bit closer (Mono/Di), by 12 no one knows who belongs to what (Mono/Mono), and when the clock strikes 13 we are all just stuck (Conjoined)"

Thyroid in Pregnancy, Thyroid Disease and Storm

The thyroid changes in pregnancy are affected primarily by β-hCG as shown in the bottom right of the drawing. Also, the fetal thyroid is not producing thyroid hormone until around 12 weeks of gestation. Thus, the management of the maternal thyroid status is imperative for proper fetal development.

The thyroid hormones Thyroxine (T4) and Triiodothyronine (T3) can cross the placenta along with iodine. The crossing of these substances are important for fetal growth and development.

Thyroid Storm is a hyper-metabolic state brought on by T4 Excess and is considered an emergency.

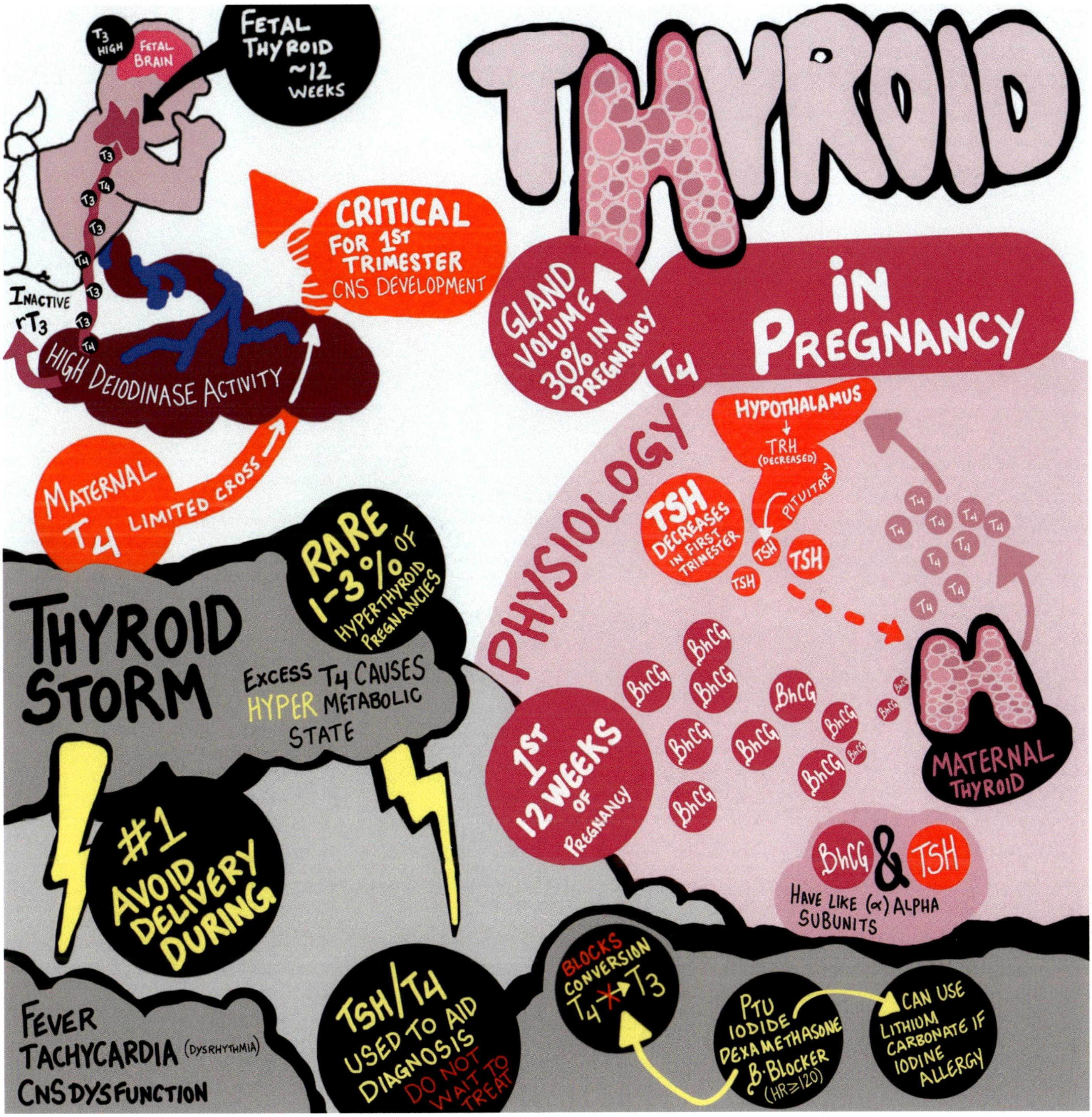

THYROID
IN PREGNANCY
T3 HIGH
FETAL BRAIN
FETAL THYROID ~12 WEEKS
CRITICAL FOR 1ST TRIMESTER CNS DEVELOPMENT
INACTIVE rT3
HIGH DEIODINASE ACTIVITY
MATERNAL T4 LIMITED CROSS
GLAND VOLUME ↑ 30% IN PREGNANCY
T4
PHYSIOLOGY
HYPOTHALAMUS
TRH (DECREASED)
PITUITARY
TSH DECREASES IN FIRST TRIMESTER
TSH
BhCG
1ST 12 WEEKS OF PREGNANCY
MATERNAL THYROID
BhCG & TSH
HAVE LIKE (α) ALPHA SUBUNITS
THYROID STORM
RARE 1-3% OF HYPERTHYROID PREGNANCIES
EXCESS T4 CAUSES HYPER METABOLIC STATE
#1 AVOID DELIVERY DURING
FEVER
TACHYCARDIA (DYSRHYTHMIA)
CNS DYSFUNCTION
TSH/T4 USED TO AID DIAGNOSIS
DO NOT WAIT TO TREAT
BLOCKS CONVERSION T4 ✕ T3
PTU
IODIDE
DEXAMETHASONE
β-BLOCKER (HR≥120)
CAN USE LITHIUM CARBONATE IF IODINE ALLERGY

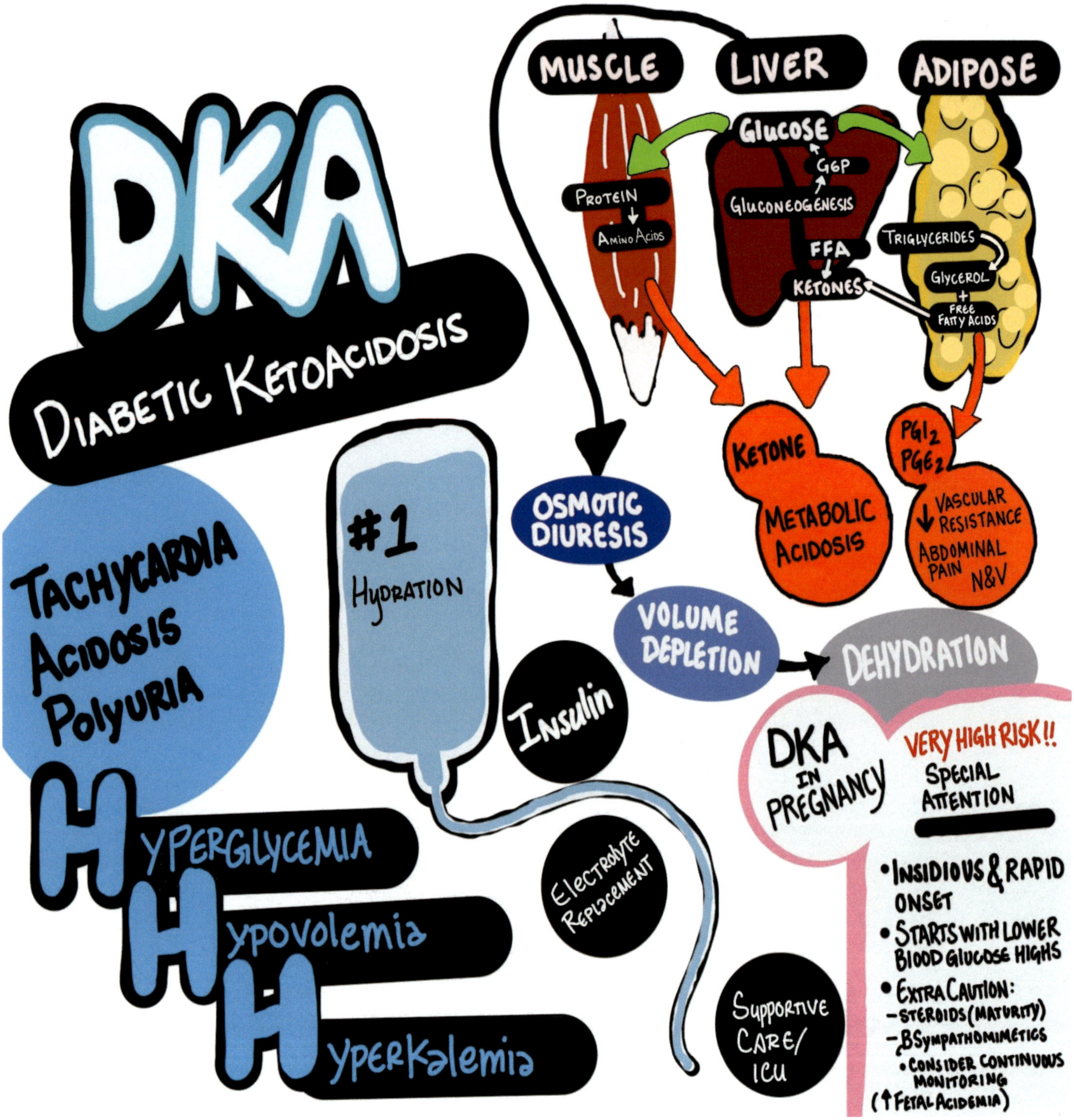

Diabetic Ketoacidosis and Pregnancy Tips

Diabetic Ketoacidosis, or DKA, is another medical emergency. This state can be caused by infection, stress or insulin deficiency. Once the body has entered into this process, it undergoes lipolysis, ketogenesis and gluconeognesis in an attempt to "feed" the cells that are sending out signals that they are not receiving glucose due to an absence of insulin. However, the above processes result in an increased glucose state (usually blood glucose > 250 mg/dL). This state leads to an osmotic diuresis and dehydration. Extra caution should be taken with the pregnant patient (as depicted in the lower right corner of the drawing) when dealing with DKA.

Preterm Birth and Pregnancy of Uncertain Viability

The question of viability and preterm delivery are all every day questions and scenarios for the Obstetrician. You should be familiar with and know these topics very well.

Preterm birth in the United States currently affects approximately 1 in 10 infants born. Of course, there are serious sequelae and significantly increases costs in the healthcare system.

Make sure you understand when to use progesterone (IM or Vaginal) or Cerclage, as these are very common board questions.

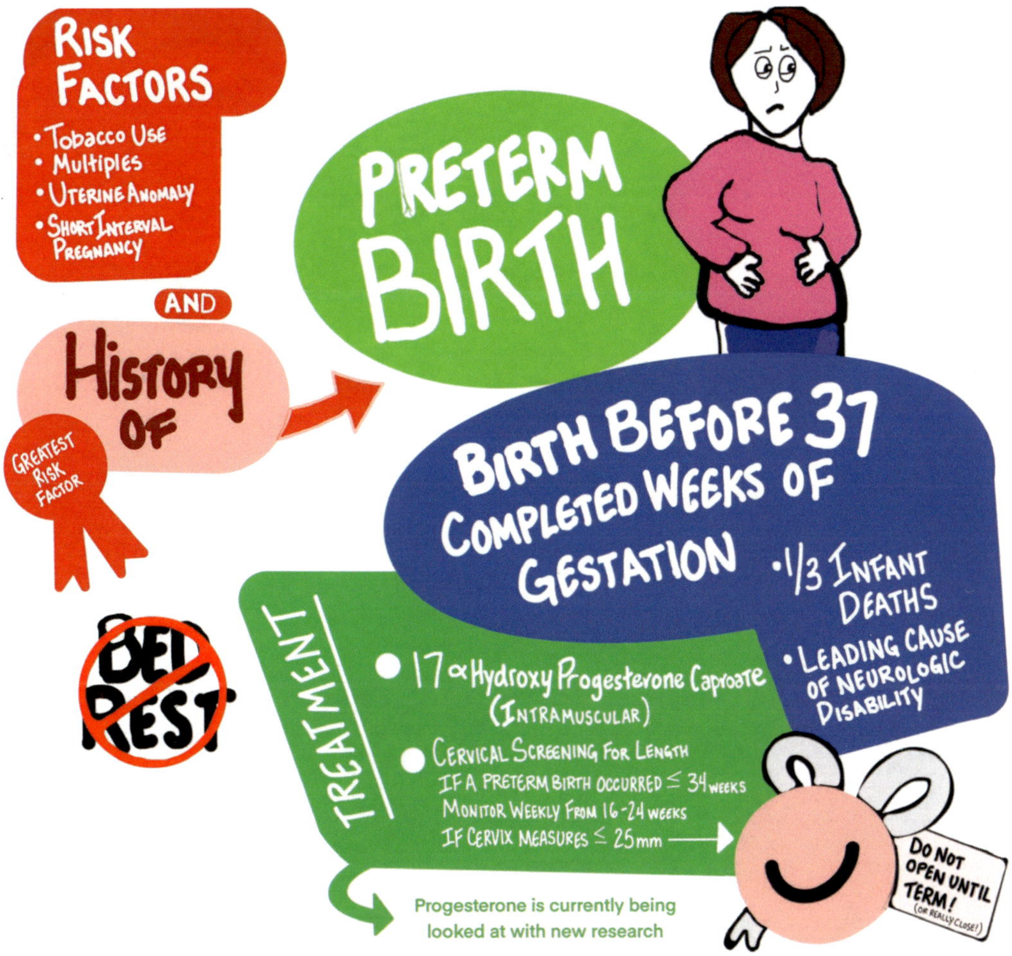

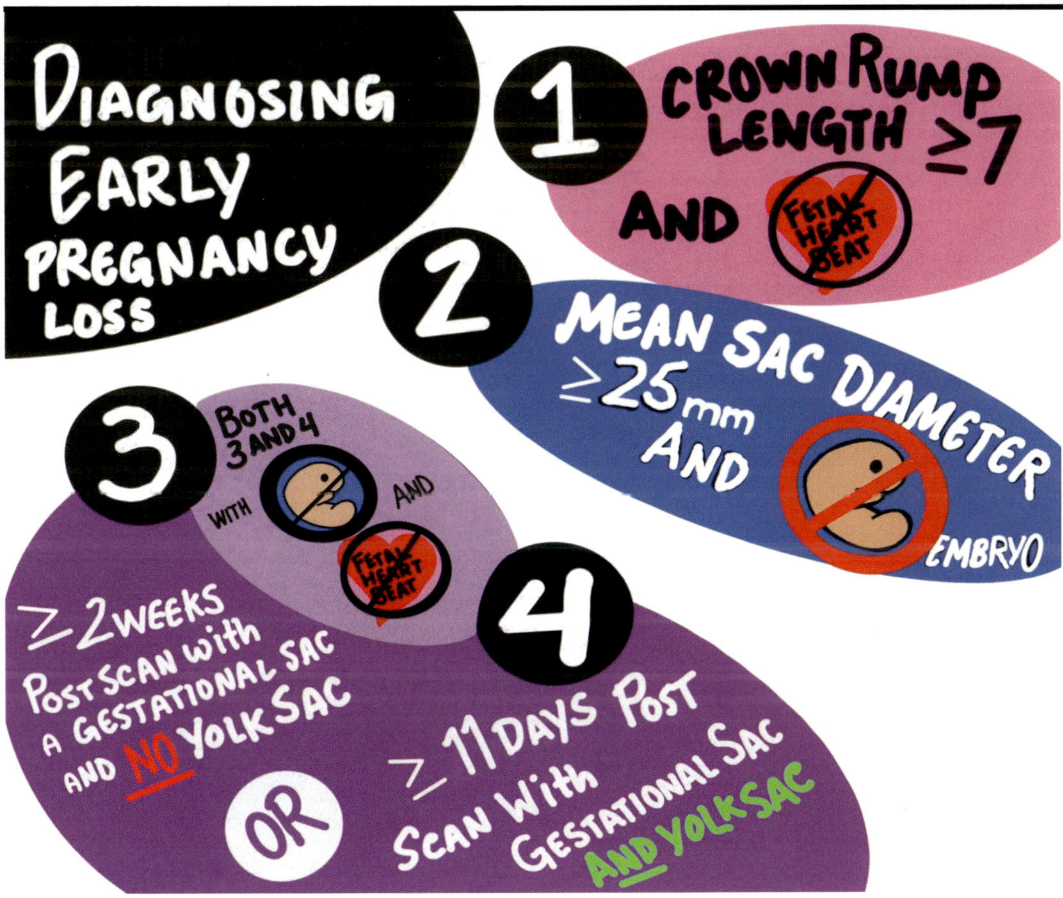

About every third call you will receive from the emergency room will be about early pregnancy loss and viability (as you have experienced in residency).

However, knowing this material is vital so we never miss a viable pregnancy or call a loss too early.

Make sure you can diagnose using each of the criteria (1, 2, 3 and 4 in the drawing) as the answer foils are commonly a variation of each of them, or all of them together.

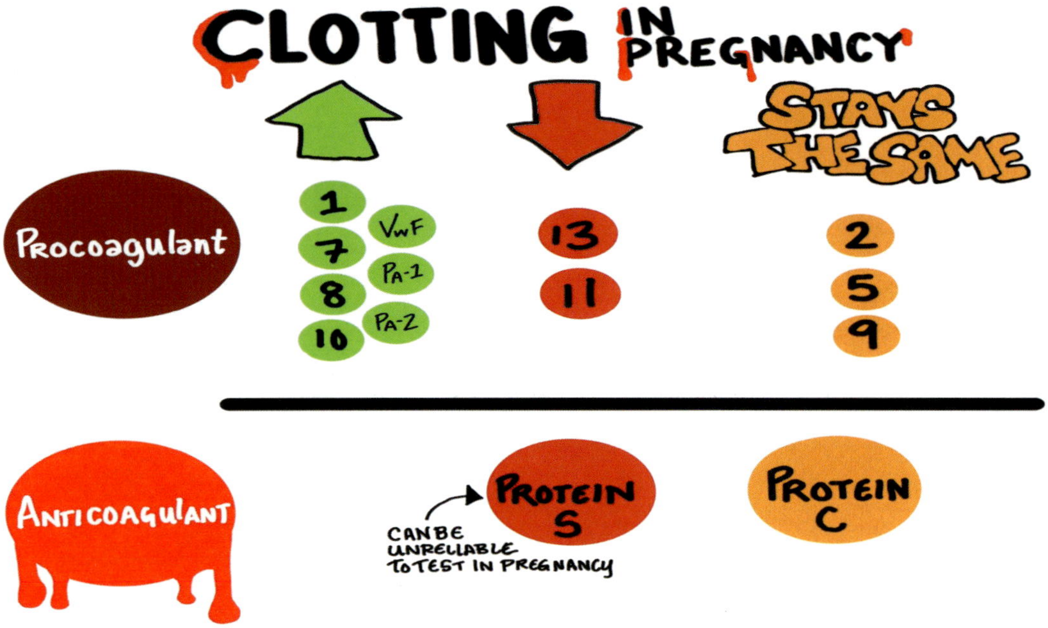

Thrombophilias and Clotting in Pregnancy

Clotting and blood disorders in the pregnant patient is one of the highest yield obstetric topics and are often complex questions on board exams. The focus is often on diagnosis and treatment. This will help summarize these important topics.

THROMBOPHILIA TREATMENT

RISK	ANTEPARTUM	POSTPARTUM
MODERATE HIGH RISK THROMBOPHILIA NO HISTORY DVT/VTE: AntiThrombin 3 Double Hetero PG20210A Homozygous FVL Homozygous PG20210A	Prophylactic Lovenox	Prophylactic Lovenox (6 weeks)
LOW WITHOUT VTE Low Risk NO HISTORY VTE: HETERO FVL HETERO PG20210A Protein C Proteins	Prophylactic Lovenox OR Surveillance	Prophylactic Lovenox OR Surveillance
APLAS WITH VTE	Prophylaxis OR Surveillance AND ASA	Surveillance

ONLY!! IF NO ADDITIONAL RISK FACTORS =
- 1° RELATIVE HISTORY THROMBOTIC EPISODE ≤50 yo
- OBESITY
- IMMOBILIZED

DOSE

LMWH	Mg
Prophylactic	40 DAY
Intermediate	40 BID

HEPARIN Trimester	Units (BID)
First	5,000-7,500
Second	7,500-10,000
Third	10,000

Reliability and Testing for Thrombophilia

	Method of Testing	When Pregnant	Acute Thrombosis	On Anti-Coag Rx
Antithrombin 3	Antithrombin Activity (<60%)	✓	⊘	⊘
Factor V Leiden	Activated Protein C Assay (Abnormal = DNA)	✓	✓	⊘ Assay ✓ DNA
PG 20210A Heterozygous	DNA Analysis	✓	✓	✓
Protein C Deficiency	Protein C Activity (<60%)	✓	⊘	⊘
Protein S Deficiency	Free Ag: Non-Pregnant <55% 2nd Trimester <30% 3rd Trimester <24%	? Levels to test ↓ with increasing gestation causing lower reliability. Adjusted scale suggested	⊘	⊘

Remember that testing for most thrombophilias can be altered by different states, such as, an active thrombotic event and when a patient is being treated with an anticoagulant. In the "method of testing" column, you will notice Factor V Leiden has an Activated Protein C Assay. If this testing shows an abnormal result, the patient should then undergo DNA testing as the next step.

Cardiac and Pulmonary Disorders of Pregnancy

With 1 in 3,000 women affected by the pathology of Peripartum Cardiomyopathy and its possible morbidity and mortality, it is a popular topic for testing. The actual pathophysiology is still being studied for this condition, however, strong correlation has been found with Prolactin, Oxidative Stress, Vascular Endothelial Growth Factor (VEGF) and Soluble FMS-Like Tyrosine Kinase.

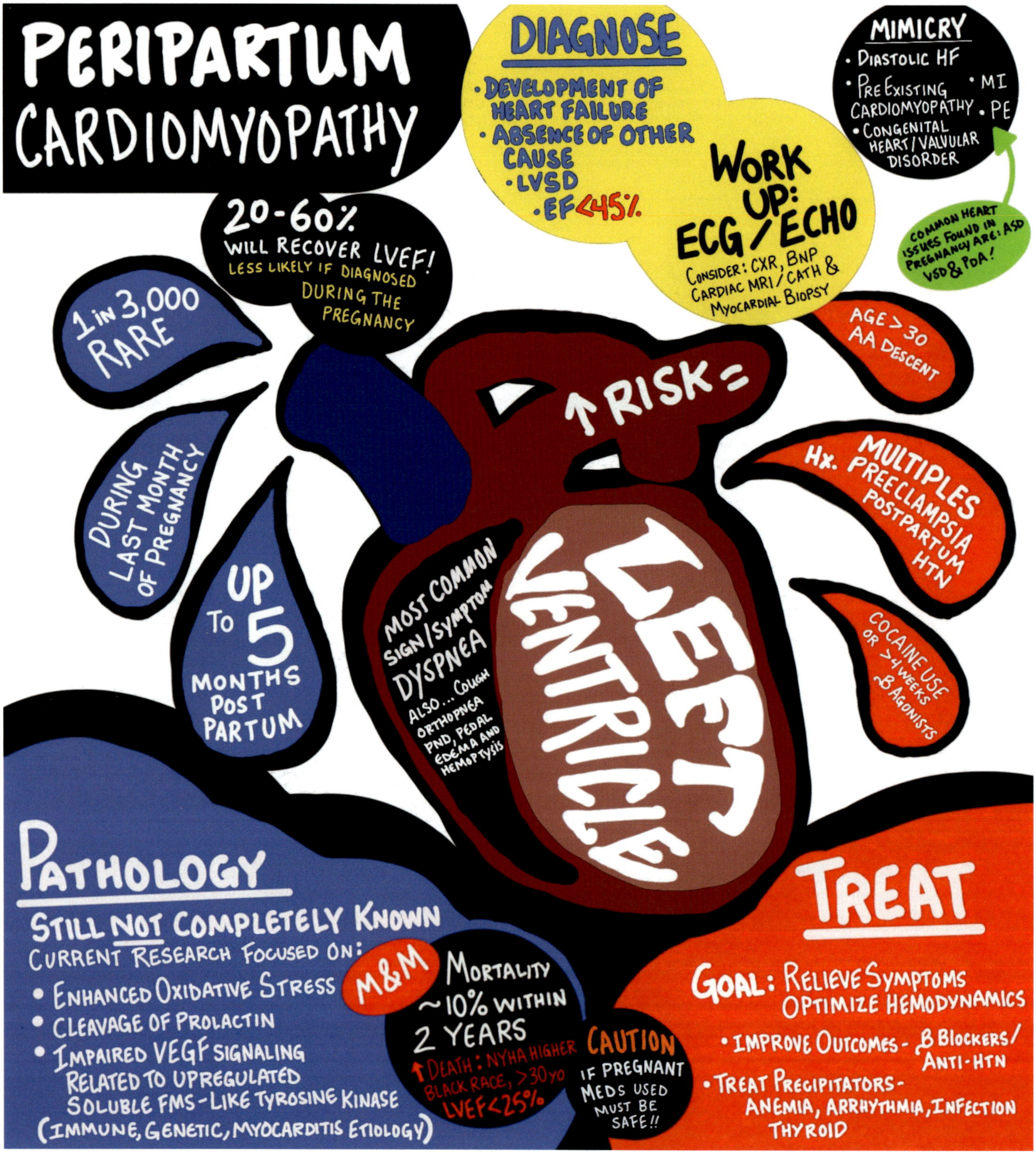

PERIPARTUM CARDIOMYOPATHY
DIAGNOSE
• DEVELOPMENT OF HEART FAILURE
• ABSENCE OF OTHER CAUSE
• LVSD
• EF<45%
WORK UP: ECG / ECHO
CONSIDER: CXR, BNP CARDIAC MRI / CATH & MYOCARDIAL BIOPSY
MIMICRY
• DIASTOLIC HF
• PRE EXISTING CARDIOMYOPATHY
• MI
• PE
• CONGENITAL HEART / VALVULAR DISORDER
COMMON HEART ISSUES FOUND IN PREGNANCY ARE: ASD VSD & PDA!
20-60% WILL RECOVER LVEF! LESS LIKELY IF DIAGNOSED DURING THE PREGNANCY
1 IN 3,000 RARE
DURING LAST MONTH OF PREGNANCY
UP TO 5 MONTHS POST PARTUM
↑ RISK =
AGE > 30 AA DESCENT
Hx. MULTIPLES PREECLAMPSIA POSTPARTUM HTN
COCAINE USE OR >4 WEEKS β AGONISTS
MOST COMMON SIGN/SYMPTOM DYSPNEA
ALSO... COUGH ORTHOPNEA PND, PEDAL EDEMA AND HEMOPTYSIS
LEFT VENTRICLE
PATHOLOGY
STILL NOT COMPLETELY KNOWN
CURRENT RESEARCH FOCUSED ON:
• ENHANCED OXIDATIVE STRESS
• CLEAVAGE OF PROLACTIN
• IMPAIRED VEGF SIGNALING RELATED TO UPREGULATED SOLUBLE FMS-LIKE TYROSINE KINASE
(IMMUNE, GENETIC, MYOCARDITIS ETIOLOGY)
M&M
MORTALITY ~10% WITHIN 2 YEARS
↑ DEATH: NYHA HIGHER BLACK RACE, >30YO LVEF<25%
CAUTION IF PREGNANT MEDS USED MUST BE SAFE!!
TREAT
GOAL: RELIEVE SYMPTOMS OPTIMIZE HEMODYNAMICS
• IMPROVE OUTCOMES - β BLOCKERS/ ANTI-HTN
• TREAT PRECIPITATORS - ANEMIA, ARRHYTHMIA, INFECTION THYROID

8 CARDIAC CONTRAINDICATIONS FOR PREGNANCY

- MARFAN'S SYNDROME WITH AORTIC ROOT ≥4 cm
- PULMONARY HYPERTENSION (PAP > 25 mmHg)
- CARDIOMYOPATHY WITH HEART FAILURE (EF < 30%)
- HISTORY OF PERIPARTUM CARDIOMYOPATHY
- BICUSPID AORTIC VALVE WITH AORTIC ROOT DILATATION (≥4-5 cm)
- SEVERE MITRAL STENOSIS
- SEVERE SYMPTOMATIC AORTIC STENOSIS
- NATIVE SEVERE COARCTATION

Amniotic Fluid Embolism

Rare yet catastrophic OB emergency

2-7 cases per 100,000 births

Possible Patho?

Amniotic fluid enters mom's circulation → inflammatory mediators → anaphylactic reaction

Usual Course

Most commonly during the labor or immediate postpartum period (as late as 48h)

Hallmark: Cardiovascular collapse

Signs and Symptoms

- Acute dyspnea
- Cyanosis
- Tachycardia

Labor Events ↑ Risk

Think: fast and furious

- Precipitous
- Abruption
- IOL
- Uterine rupture
- Cervical laceration

Management

#1 Early recognition and management with anesthesia team

- Activate massive blood transfusion protocol
- Prepare OR, ICU & interventional radiology
- Focus on airway & circulation support
- Balance coagulopathy !!

Three Main Phases

1. Pulmonary/systemic hypertension
2. ↓SVR and LV stroke work index
3. Lung injury & coagulopathy

- Hysterectomy may be needed
- Expedite delivery
- Consider factor 7 usage

Increased Risk

- AMA
- Polyhydramnios
- Multip
- Diabetes
- PreE/Eclampsia

Pulmonary Embolus

Signs/Symptoms

- **Dyspnea** with:
  - Tachycardia
  - Hypoxia
  - Pleuritic chest pain
  - Cough

Most common. However, found to greatly vary and be nonspecific

Well's Criteria

Can assist with unclear clinical assessment

Score >4.0 positive result (PTE likely)

Diagnosis

CT pulmonary angiography (most available standard)

SN: 83% SP: 96%

Moderate suspicion: D-dimer, US Doppler

Management

- Oxygenation (intubation)
- Fluids & vasopressors
- Anticoagulation !!!

Hepatitis B and the Pregnant Patient

Understanding the many states of serology that occurs with hepatitis B is extremely important for women's health and the pregnant patient. Commonly asked states on exams are the "Vaccinated" state and the "Acute" versus "Chronic" state.

The "Acute" state is recognized by the presence of Anti-HBc IgM. The drawing depicts the **"M"** from Ig**M** fitting into the shape of the **"A"** from **A**cute. The "Chronic" state shows the **"G"** from Ig**G** and the "**C**" from **C**hronic fitting together. This is a memory trick to help determine between an Acute or Chronic State. Both states have HBs Antigen and the HBe Antigen present, so alone they will not help to distinguish the state of the patient. When using the IgM and IgG you should be able to determine which state the patient is in.

Important pregnancy related Hepatitis B information from the ACOG Practice Bulletin #86 includes:

- All pregnant women should be screened with HBsAg
- Newborns born to infected women should have HBIG and Hepatitis B vaccine within 12 hours of birth
- Women at risk for contracting Hepatitis B should receive the vaccination, even when pregnant
- If a woman is HBsAg positive, or if chronically infected, and the infant has received HBIG and vaccination; breastfeeding is NOT contraindicated.
- Women acutely infected in the first trimester are less likely (10%) to vertically transmit than if the transmission occurs during the third trimester (80-90%). Congenital acquired infection has a much higher risk of lifetime complications (25-30%) for the infant compared to adult acquired (5-10%

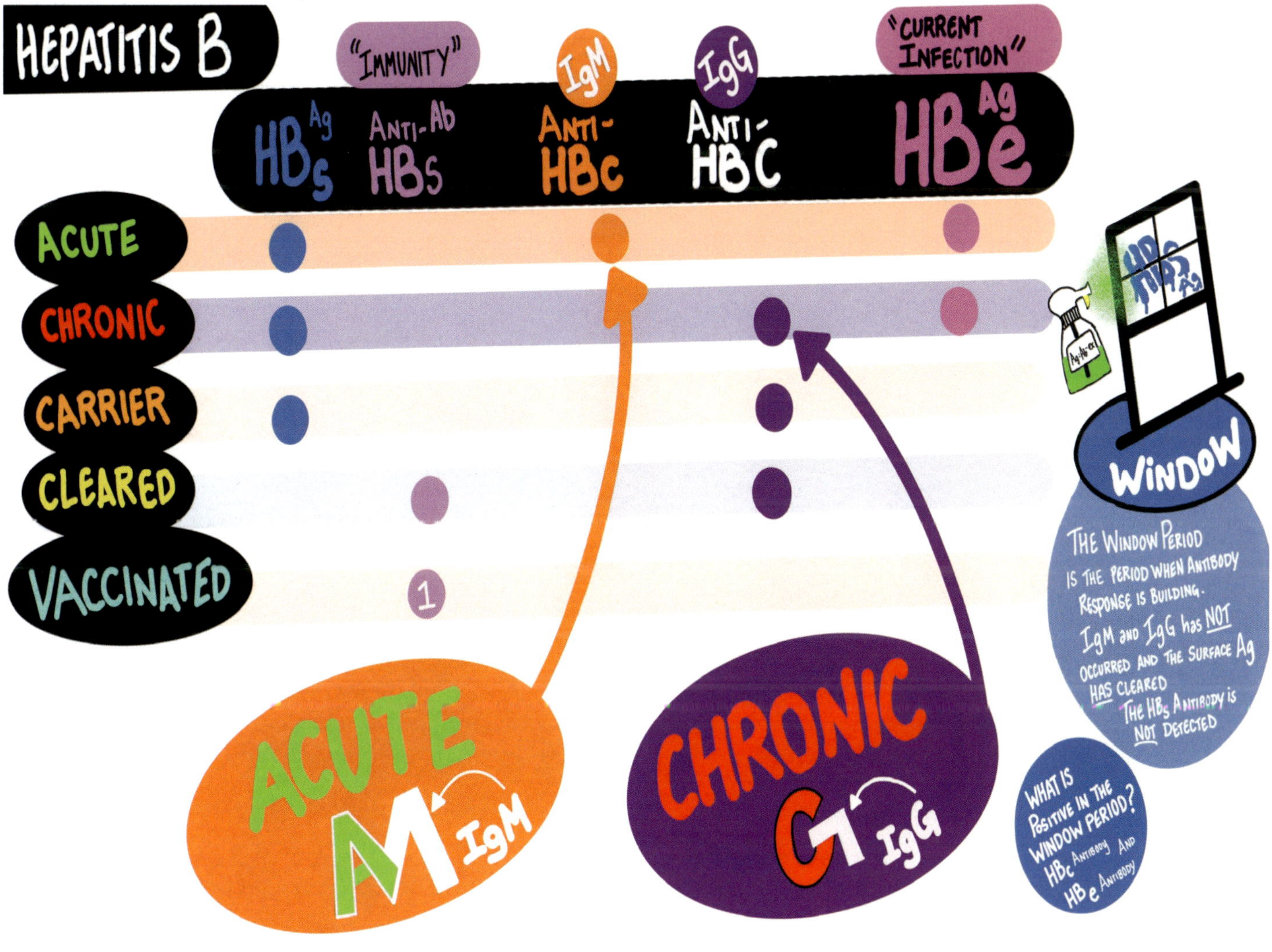

Birth Related Nerve Injuries

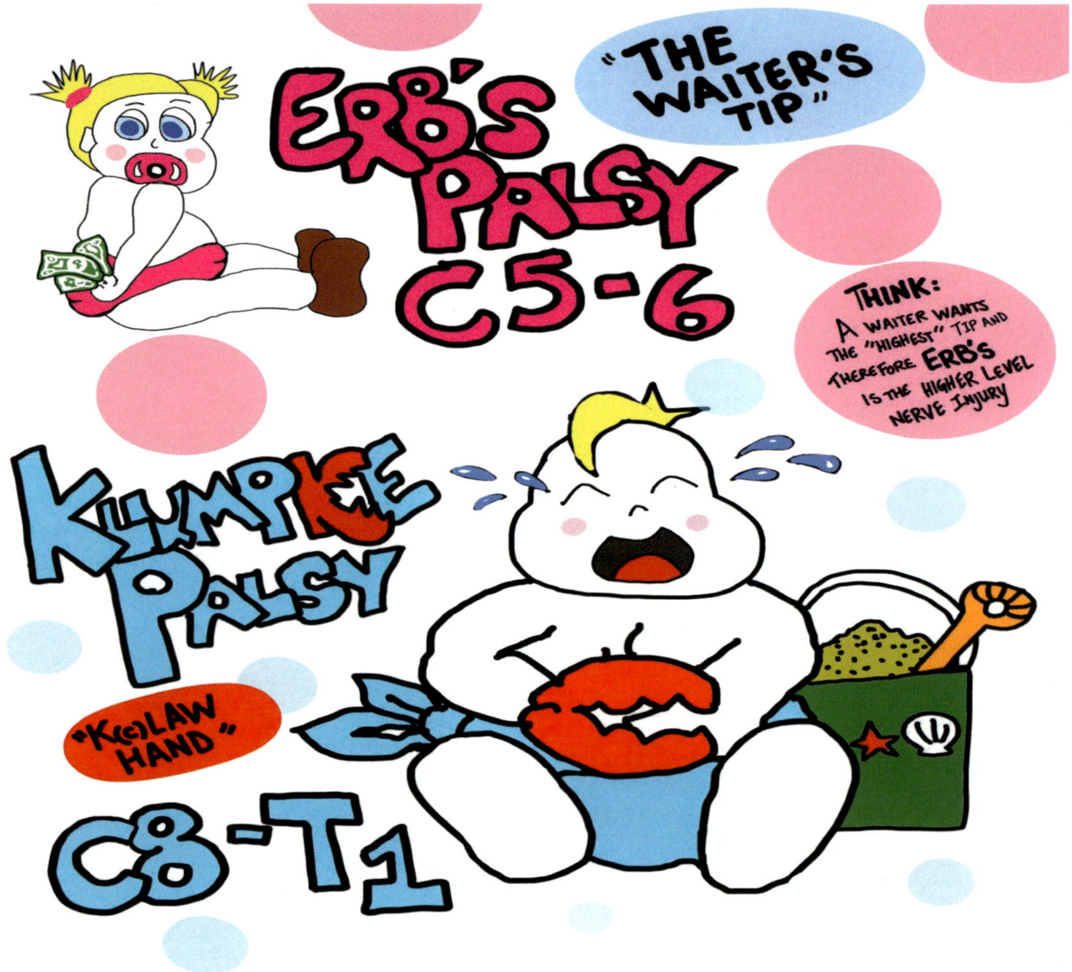
ERB'S PALSY C5-6
"THE WAITER'S TIP"
THINK: A WAITER WANTS THE "HIGHEST" TIP AND THEREFORE ERB'S IS THE HIGHER LEVEL NERVE INJURY
KLUMPKE PALSY
"K(C)LAW HAND"
C8-T1

Nerve injuries are devastating to mothers after birthing their infants. The most common reason these injuries occur is related to fetal macrosomia and those conditions resulting in shoulder dystocia. Most studies of infants with brachial plexus nerve injuries have shown complete resolution within 2-4 months after birth. Injuries lasting beyond this time period are uncommon. Mothers should be counseled regarding the risk of these infant injuries related to fetal macrosomia and shoulder dystocia.

APGAR

It's easy to forget some of the simplest things…

However, when it comes to APGAR just think of the baby in front of you.

A = Appearance (Color)
P = Pulse
G = Grimace
A = Activity (Tone)
R = Respirations (Cry)

Each gets a value of 0,1 or 2

Possible total of 10 (Good)

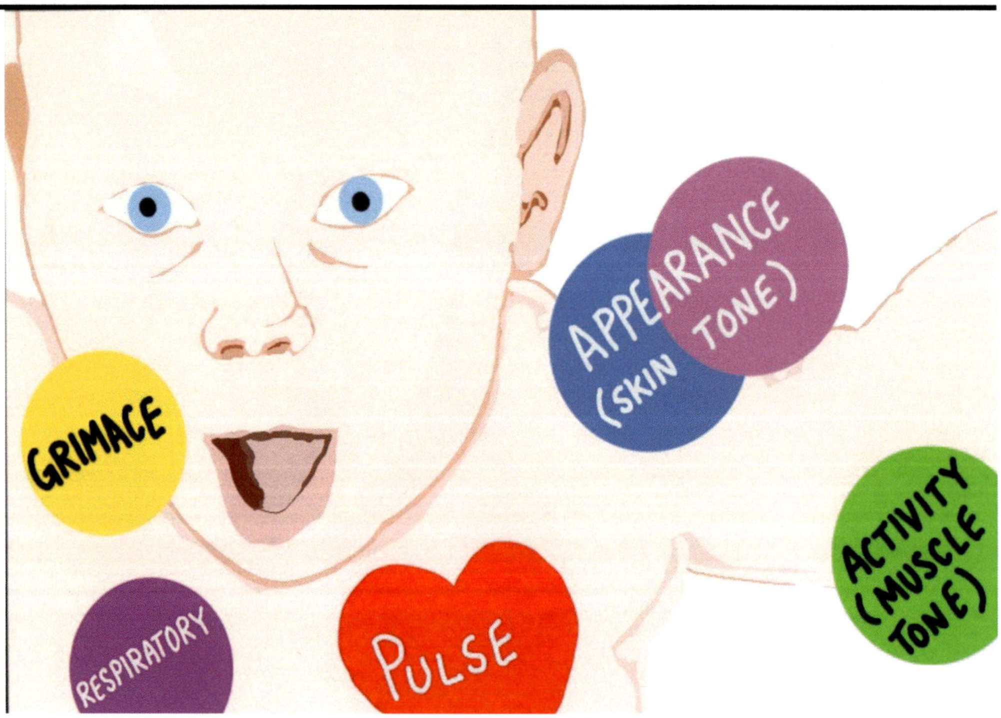

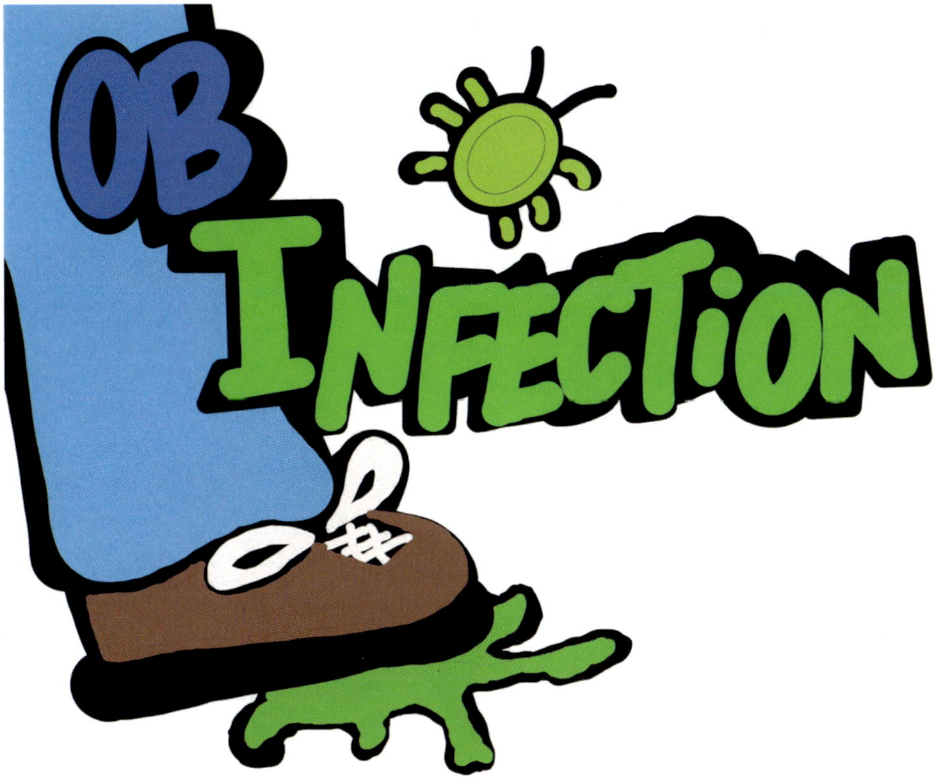

Infections in the Pregnant Patient

Whether you are shown an image of a fetal ultrasound, a newborn or just asked questions about a mother's new little one, you have to be comfortable with the signs of common OB infections.

On this table are some of the most common obstetric infections and the findings that correlate with each of them.

FINDING	RUBELLA	CMV	HSV	TOXO	SYPHILLIS
Meningoencephalitis	Blue dot	Red dot	Red dot	Red dot	Blue dot
Hepatosplenomegaly	Red dot	Red dot	Blue dot	Red dot	Red dot
Petechiae (blueberry muffin)	Blue dot	Pathognomonic	Blue dot	Yellow dot	Yellow dot
Chorioretinitis	Blue dot	Yellow dot	Yellow dot	Pathognomonic	Rare
Anemia	Yellow dot	Blue dot	Yellow dot	Red dot	Red dot
Cranial calcification	Rare	Blue dot	Yellow dot	Pathognomonic	Rare
Microcephaly	Rare	Blue dot	Yellow dot	Blue dot	Rare

= Pathognomonic

RED DOTS are common in that disease.

BLUE DOTS indicate a possible connection.

YELLOW DOTS are uncommon.

"RARE"
means rarely associated.

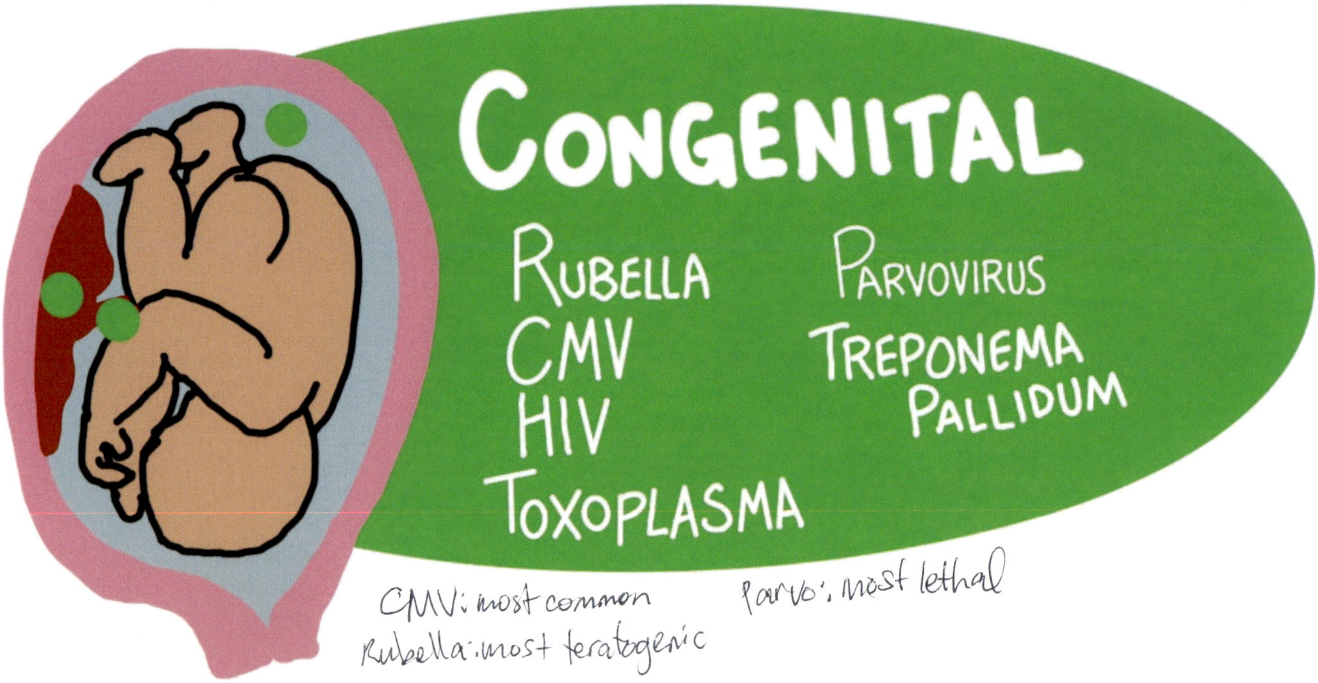

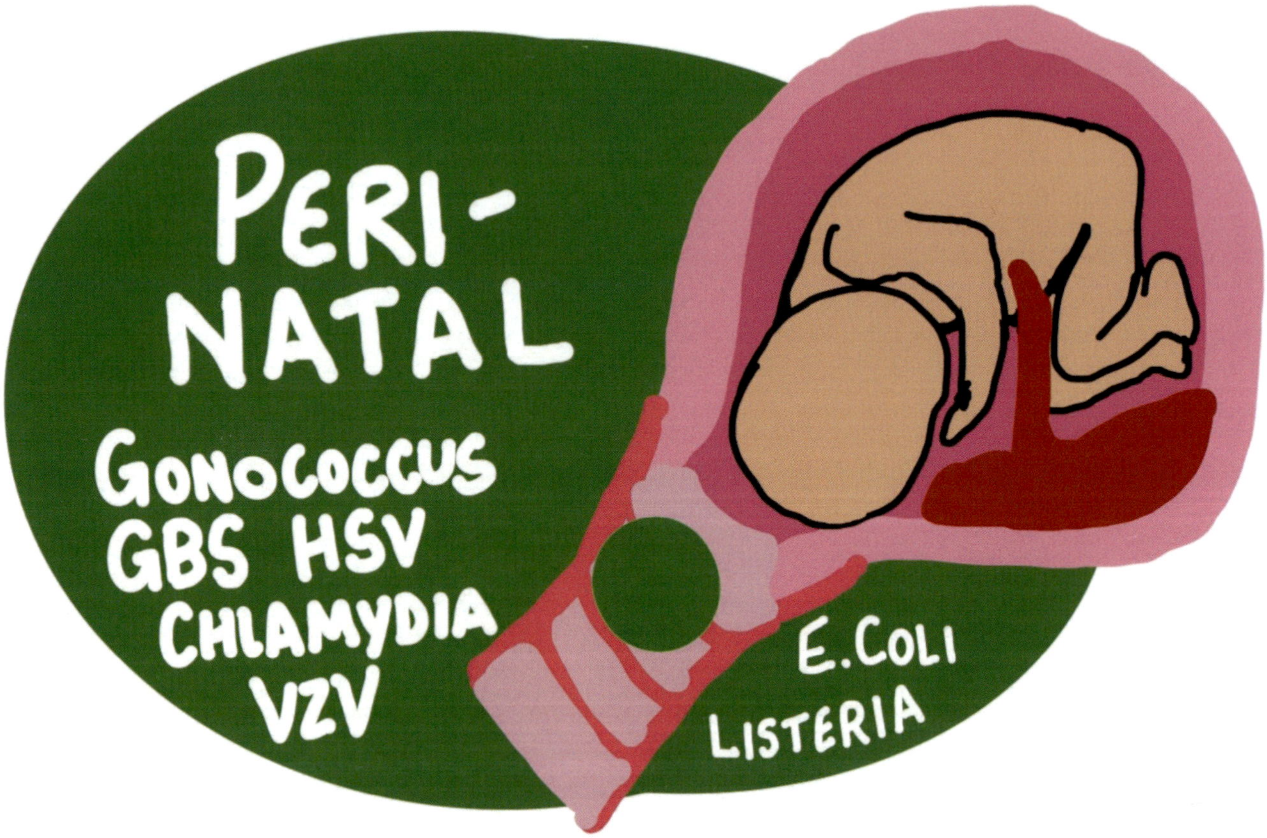

This page differentiates between congenital and perinatal infections. A small change in the wording or vignette can easily get rid of foils on your exams.

PREVENTATIVE and OFFICE

HEMOGLOBIN ELECTROPHORESIS

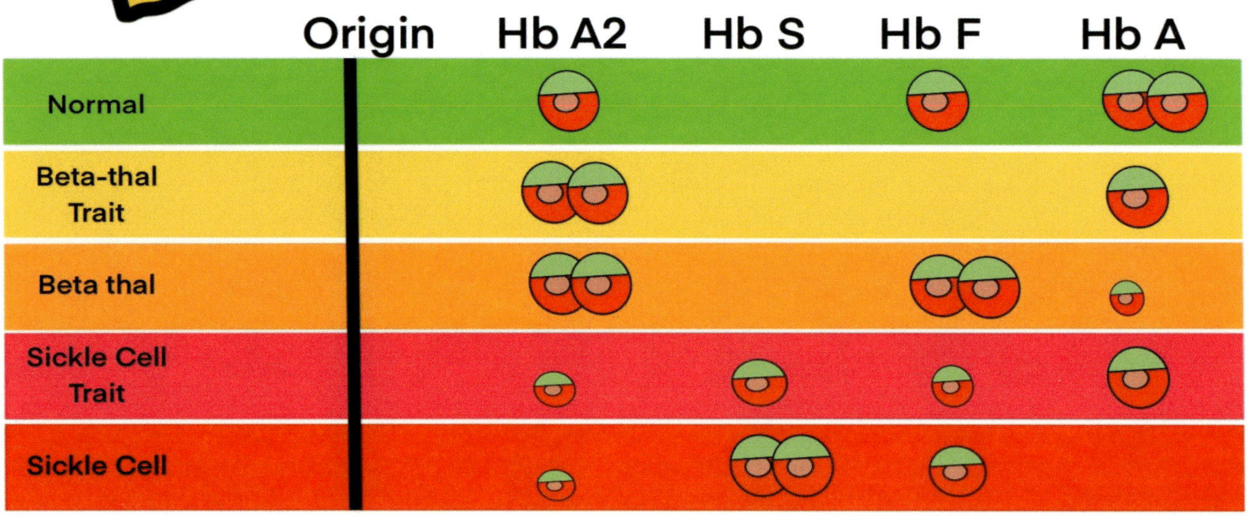

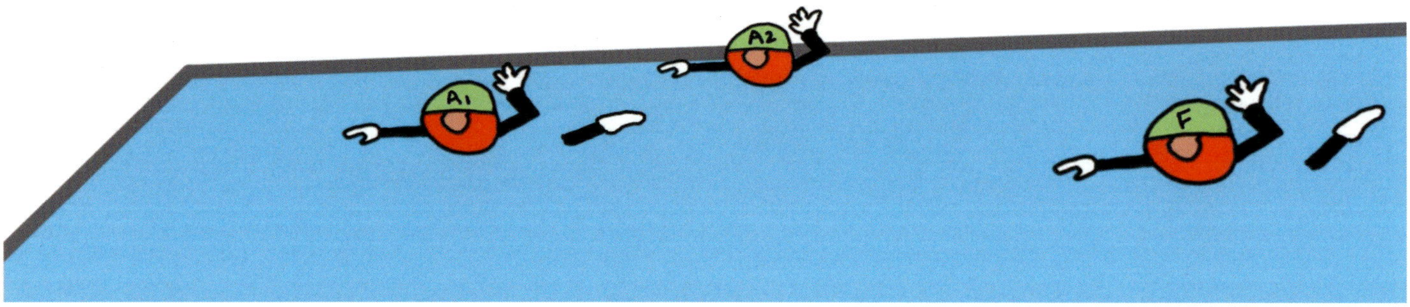

Sometimes what seems like a walk in the park, or a straight swim down a lane, can get easily confusing on an exam. Hemoglobin Electrophoresis are one of those straight forward items that ends up drowning a lot of test takers. Let's go for some high-yield facts.

First, more and larger swim capped red blood cells in a column indicates an increased presence in the normal or abnormal reading of that row. Example: a normal result (the first row) would have Hemoglobin A2 (Hb A2) and Hemoglobin F (Hb F) it would have no Hemoglobin S (Hb S) and a large amount of Hemoglobin A (Hb A).

Let's look at a commonly asked question. Which of the following would have a "normal" reading - Alpha Thalassemia or Beta Thalassemia? An easy way to remember is in the test name itself! There is no letter "A" in Hemoglobin Electrophoresis. Therefore, this study CANNOT tell you if a person has the Alpha Thalassemia as it will show up as a normal result.

Knowing your immunization facts and administration times is one of the core foundational practices in preventative care. Many women utilize their Gynecologist as their primary care providers, so we can't just "leave that up to your PCP." So, we must learn the timing of these immunizations!

The mnemonic on the syringe, "D I V H2 M2" is to help remind you of the immunizations and also help you with life long and specific timing. You can **D**el **I** **V**er the **DIV** anytime in a patient's life. Also, remember the Hepatitis Vaccine in identified high risk populations can be delivered when deemed appropriate (including during pregnancy).

Zoster is a common point of contention in primary care. There are technically two types of the vaccine available. The recombinant form known as "RZV" (Shingrix), and the live form "ZVL" (Zostavax). Think of Shingrix as "Shiny and New" as it is the preferred form. It can be given at age 50 and on and covers the patient in the more likely age range they will have shingles. Zostavax remember "let it lax". ZVL is phasing out as it was only given at ages 50-59 and did not cover as many adults when needed. RZV is now preferred over ZVL.

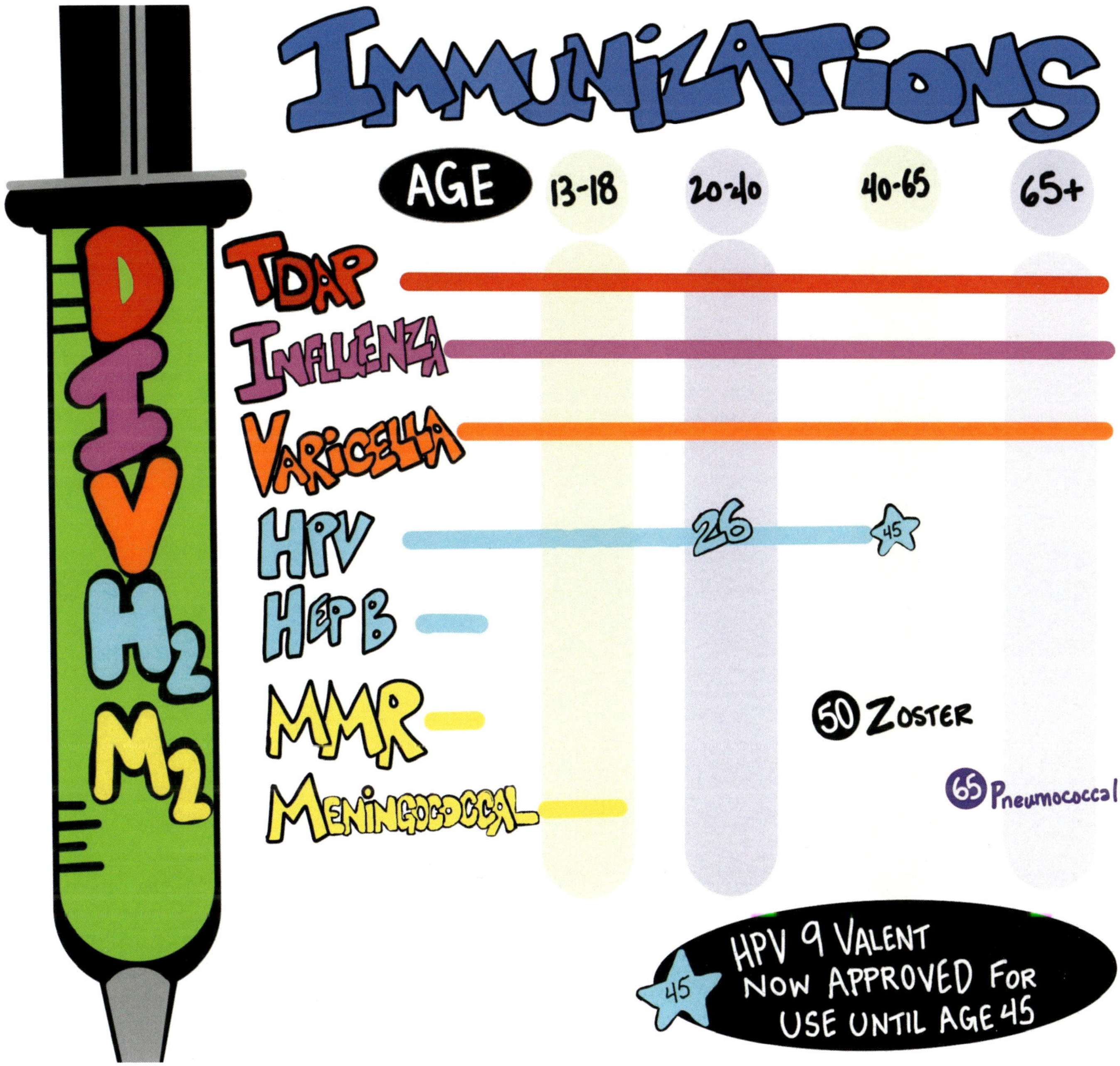

Breast Cancer Risk

The Gail Breast Risk Model is a useful clinical tool and a favorite for question writers. The biggest take home points are the variables used to determine risk: age of the individual being investigated for risk, the number of breast biopsies they have had (and presence of atypical hyperplasia), the number of primary relatives with breast cancer and when those persons (age) had their first child.

Things the Gail Breast Risk Model does NOT take into consideration are: other cancers, second degree or greater relatives and breast cancer in paternal relatives.

The Risk Model depicts High Risk as a person with a 5-year Gail Risk of >1.7%. Notice the greatest risk in the model is depicted in the drawing. This is a person with 2 or greater first degree relatives that had their first born children in their 20's. The Relative Risk of this combination is 6.8. Remember, relative risk is stated as: this person will have 6.8 times the risk of developing breast cancer than a woman without these risk factors.

Gail MH et al., J. Natl Cancer Inst. 1989;81:1879-86.

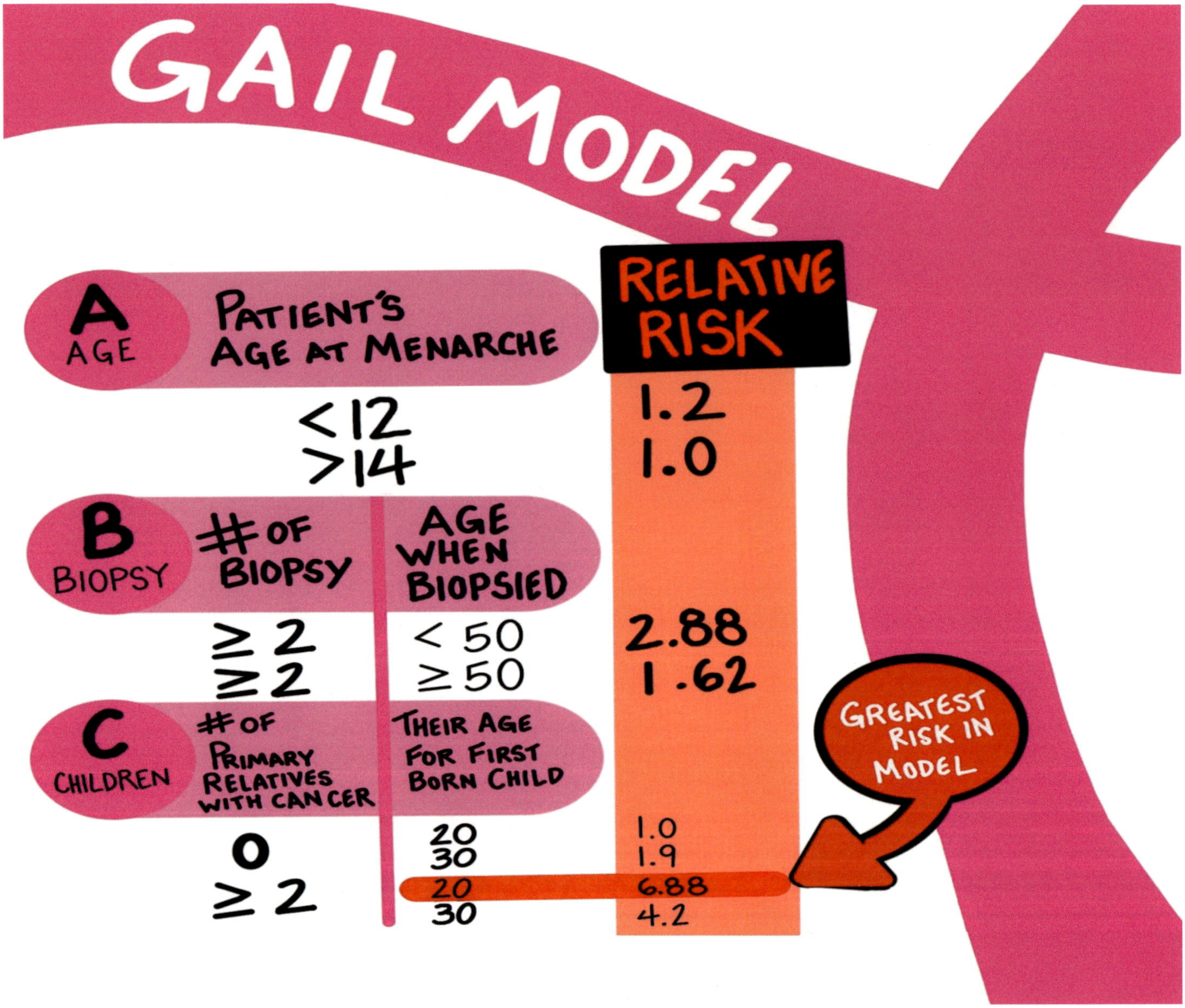

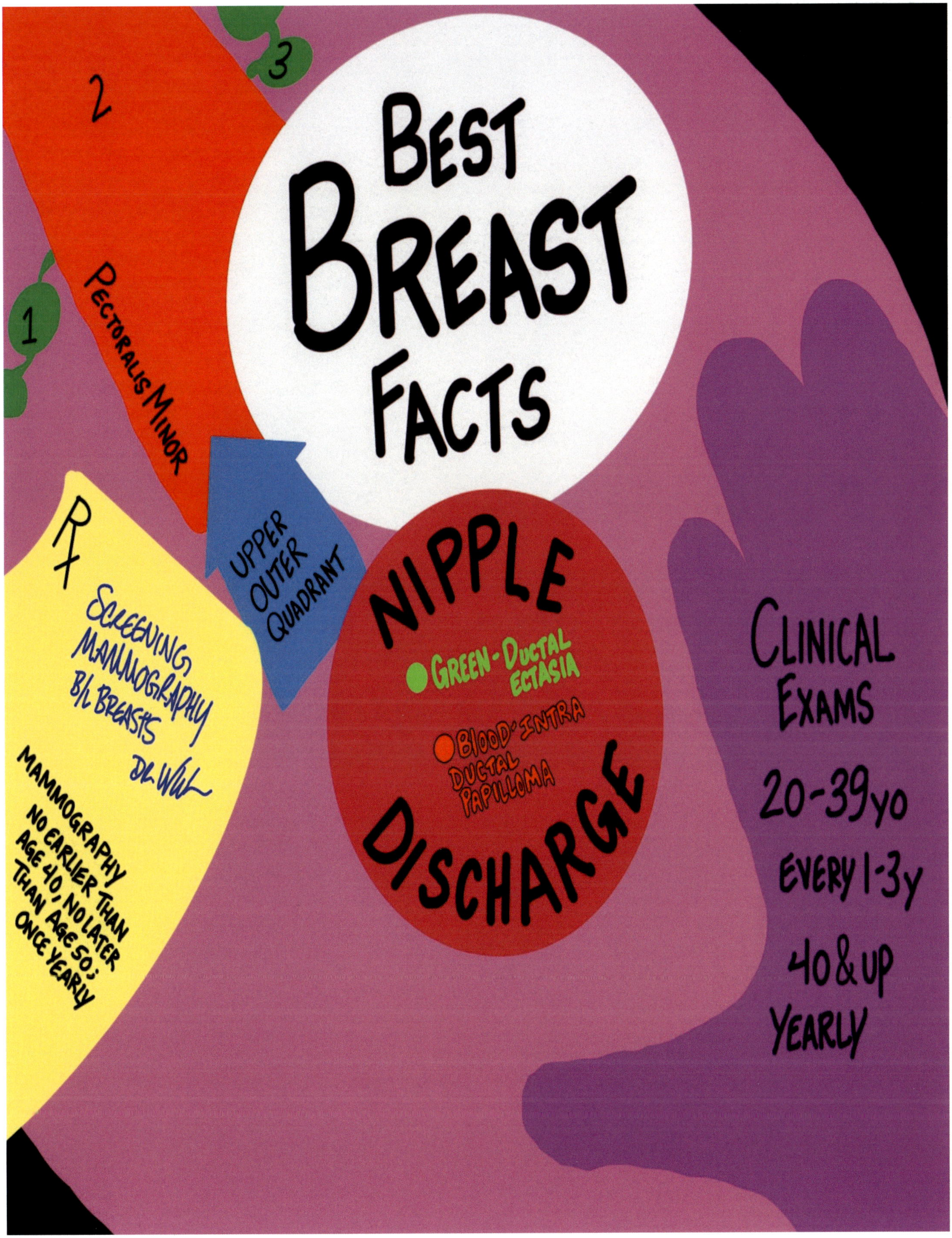
BEST BREAST FACTS
2
3
1
PECTORALIS MINOR
UPPER OUTER QUADRANT
NIPPLE DISCHARGE
GREEN - DUCTAL ECTASIA
BLOOD - INTRA DUCTAL PAPILLOMA
Rx
SCREENING MAMMOGRAPHY B/L BREASTS
DR. W
MAMMOGRAPHY NO EARLIER THAN AGE 40, NO LATER THAN AGE 50; ONCE YEARLY
CLINICAL EXAMS
20-39yo
EVERY 1-3y
40 & UP
YEARLY

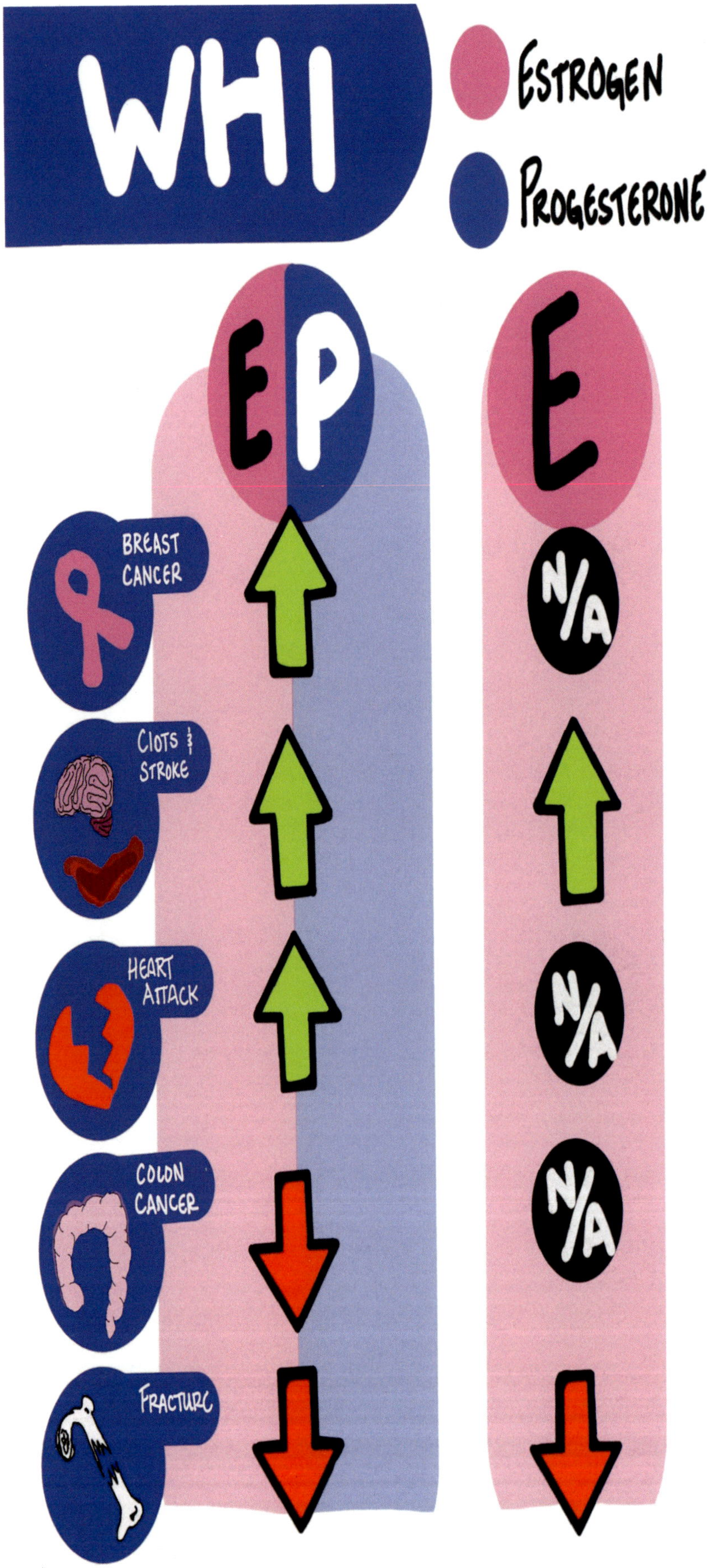

The Women's Health Initiative Study (WHI) took place in 2002 and is one of the most controversially discussed studies in Gynecology. This is why you are almost guaranteed to see a question about this study on your test!

Also, in practice you will have women that will come with questions regarding the findings that the WHI study produced. So, this knowledge is everyday practice applicable too.

The study was reexamined later and was found to include women who were much older than average for menopausal symptoms. Many of the women were also asymptomatic. However, the findings are seen as the main causes of fear and resistance to use hormone replacement therapy (HRT).

Some of the most important things to remember from this study includes:

-Estrogen and Progesterone:

INCREASE Breast Cancer, Clots, Stroke Risk and Heart Attack

-Estrogen and Progesterone:

DECREASE Colon Cancer and Bone Fractures

Absolute Contraindications for HRT:

-Breast Cancer History
-Endometrial Cancer History
-Severe Active Liver Disease
-Hypertriglyceridemia
-Thromboembolic Disorders
-Undiagnosed Vaginal Bleeding

After the WHI was published, a data set from a younger subset of women was examined, it found that composite coronary scores in the Estrogen alone arm decreased (aged 50-59). This also showed a decrease in all cause mortality in both Estrogen alone and Estrogen / Progesterone arms.

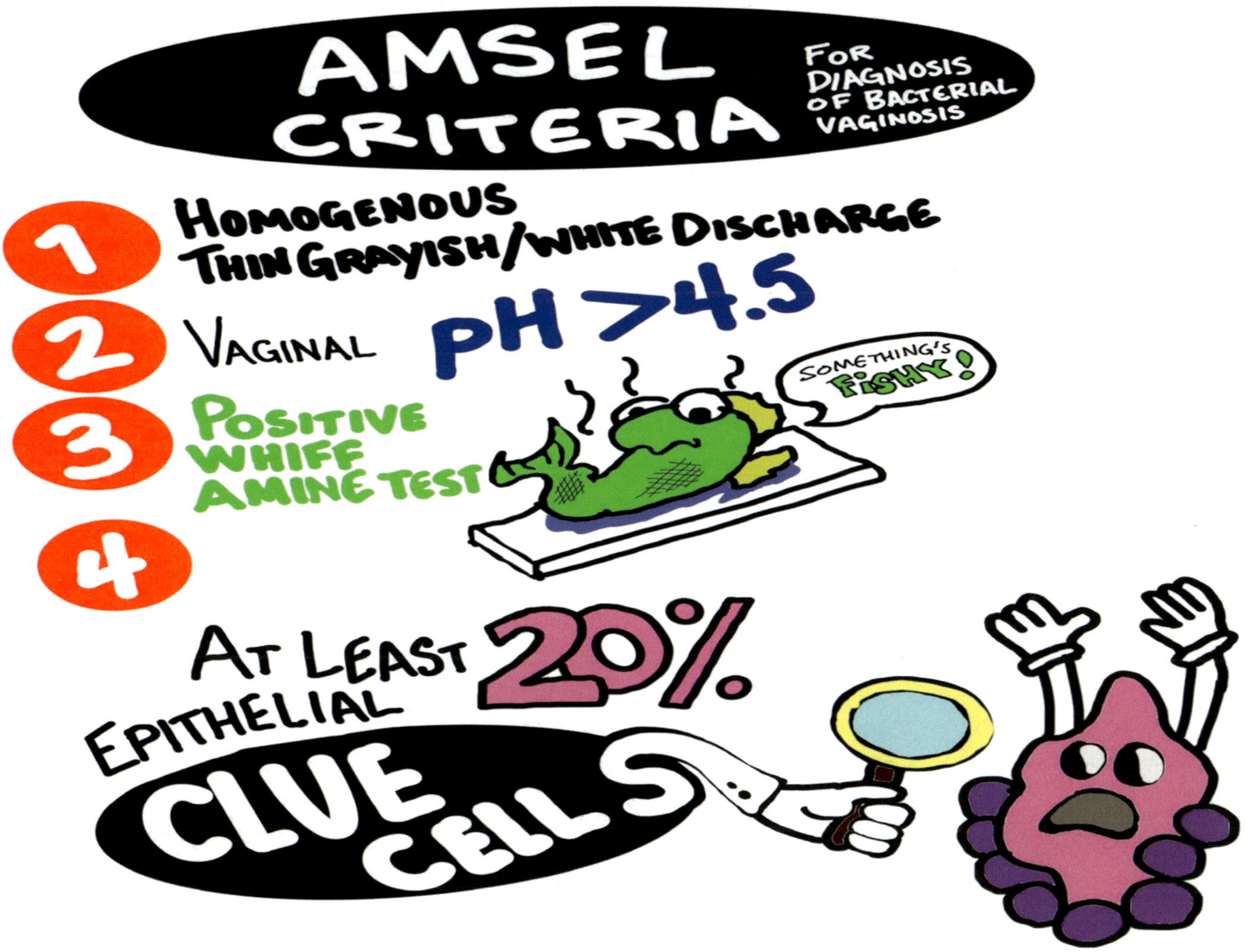

	Normal	Trichomoniasis	Candidiasis	Bacterial Vaginosis
Symptoms/ Presentation		Discharge, Itch	Itch, Discomfort, Dysuria Thick Discharge	Odor, Discharge, Itch
Vaginal Discharge	Clear to Clear-White	Frothy, Gray to Yellow-Green and malodorous	Thick, Clumpy, White “Cottage Cheese”	Homogenous, Adherent, Thin, Milky White, Malodorous “Foul” “Fishy”
Clinical Findings		Cervical Petecchie “Strawberry Cervix”	Inflammation and Erythema	
Vaginal pH	3.3 - 4.5	> 4.5	Usually ≤ 4.5	> 4.5
KOH “Whiff” Test	Negative	Often Positive	Negative	Positive
NaCl Wet Mount	Lactobacilli	Motile, Flagellated Protozoa And multiple WBC’s	Few WBC’s	Clue Cells (≥ 20%), None to Few WBC’s
Treatment		PO: Metronidazole, Tinidazole	PO: Fluconazole PV: Miconazole, Clotrimazole	PO: Metronidazole PV: Metronidazole, Clindamycin

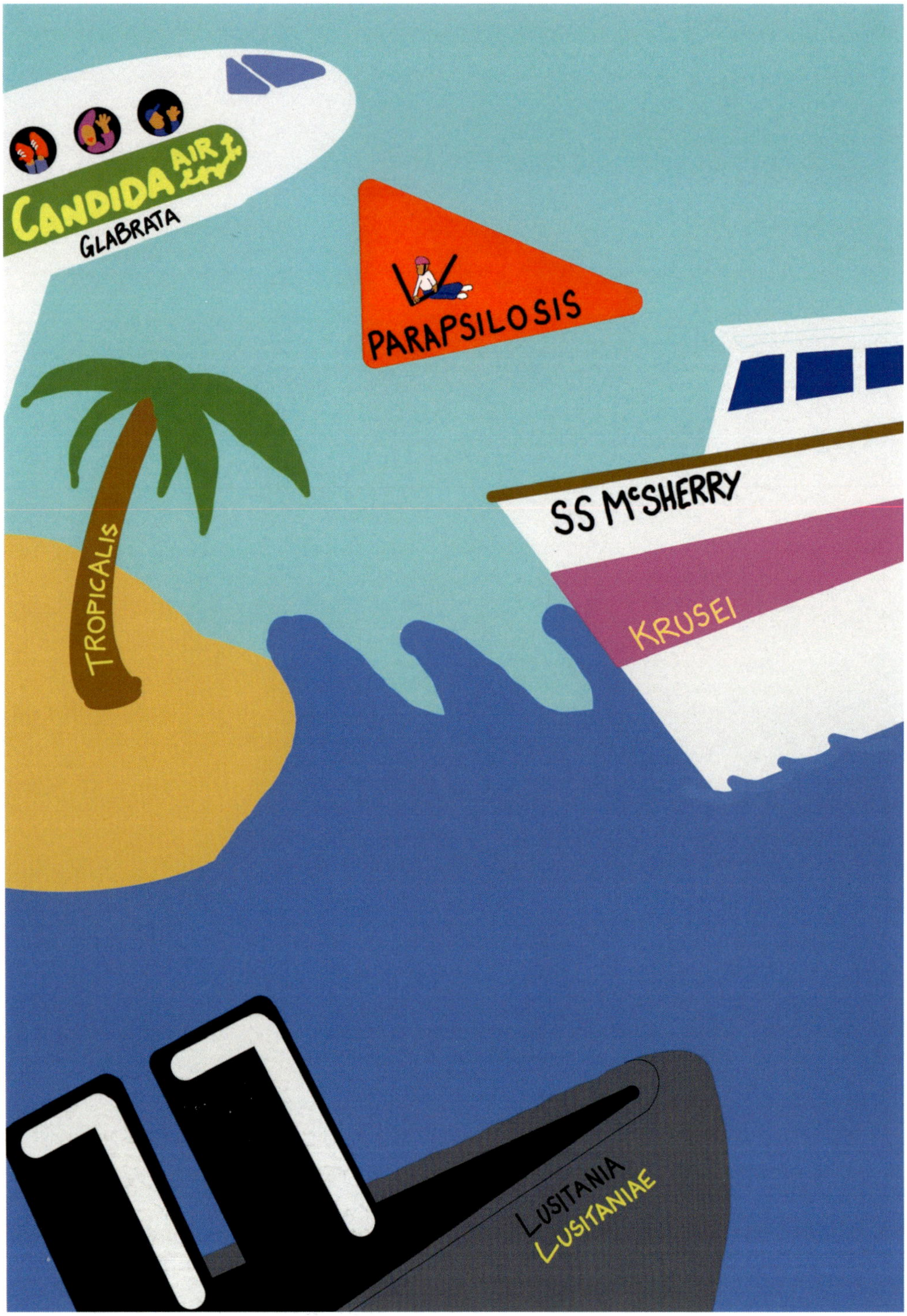

"Yeast Vacation"

(The other Candida Species)

It is important to realize that there are other forms of yeast, that will affect your patient's health. The yeast are remembered by going on a yeast vacation.

So, let's go!

First, you hop on Candida Air or **glabrata** airlines to become a "globetrotter" around the world. Of course, you want to try out a tropical location like **tropicalis.** While you are there you have to go parasailing or **parapsiolos** - ing. Next relax out on the water while taking a **krusei** on your own cruise ship. To end the perfect vacation, go scuba diving and explore the sunken World War 1 battle ship the Lusitania; which, strangely sounds and looks like **luisitaniae.** We hope you enjoyed your yeast vacation!

Here's a table for treatment of the most common isolated candida species. Important points would be albicans is treated by all formulations. The parapsilosis species is immune to Terconazole. The krusei species is the only listed that is immune to Nystatin. Knowing these important facts can easily eliminate foils on your exam.

Yeast Species	Cases by Percent	Miconozole	Fluconazole	Terconzole	Clotrimazole	Itraconazole	Nystatin
C. albicans	70%	X	X	X	X	X	X
C. glabrata	18%	X					X
C. parapsilosis	5%	X	X		X	X	X
C. krusei	2%	X			X		

Cause of Death

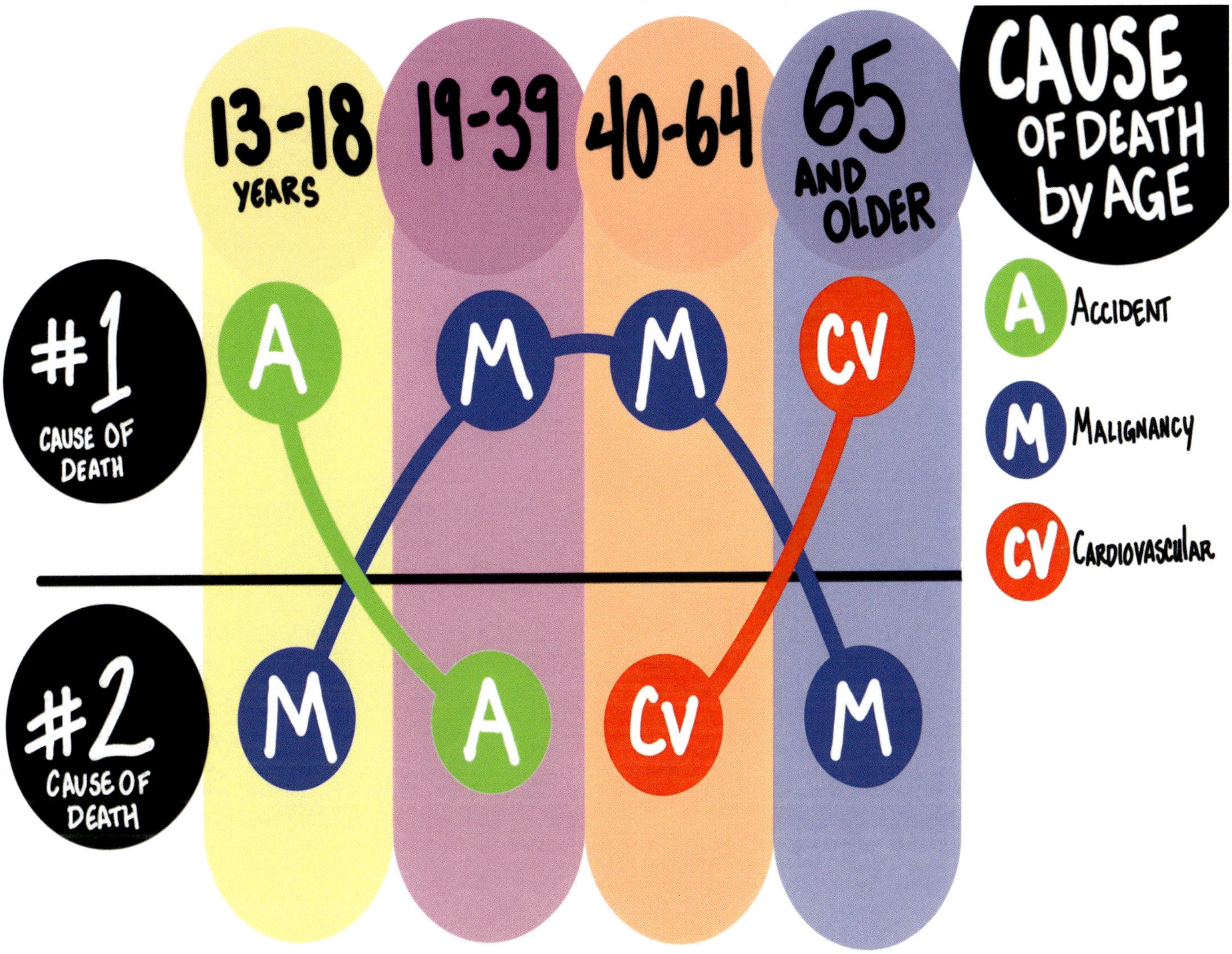

Knowing what will most likely kill your patient will help to guide her preventative care and counseling. Understanding cause of death by age is another topic on exams. This drawing will help you to better understand women's risk of death and forms a specific, and easy to recall, pattern when arranged by age. The ages in the drawing are the same ranges as the women's annual examination age categories.

Malignancy starts as the #2 cause of death for the 13-18 year old age group and then becomes the #1 cause for both the 19-39 year olds and the 40-64 year old age groups. Malignancy then becomes #2 again for the 65 years and older age group.

Accidents are the absolute #1 cause of death for the 13-18 year old age group. It becomes #2 in the 19-39 age group. Cardiovascular is the #2 cause for the 40-64 group and becomes #1 for those 65 years and older.

Learning this simple pattern will not only teach you the age ranges for annual care, but it will also answer the many common questions on examinations.

NOTES

GYNECOLOGY and SURGERY

Ureteral Injuries

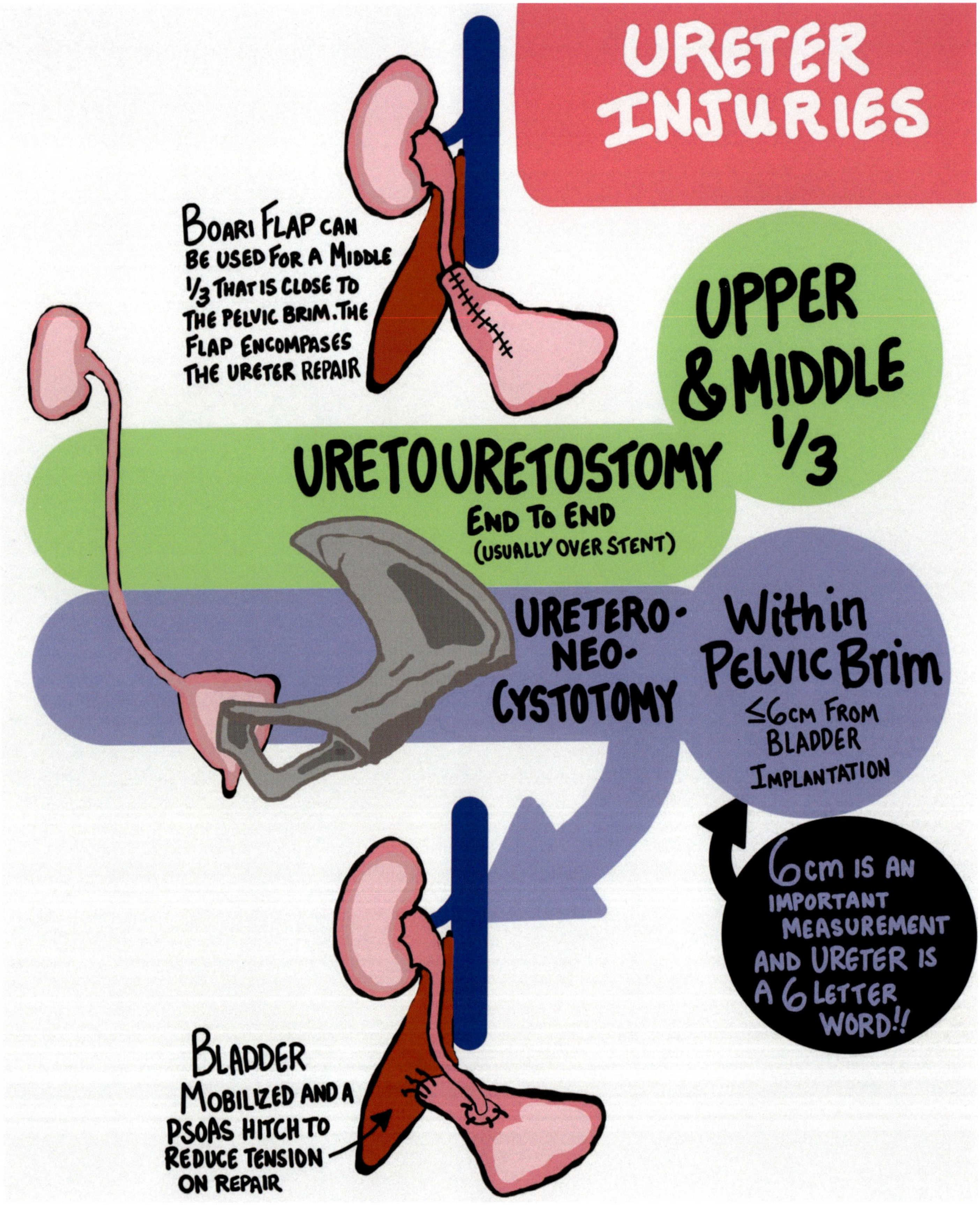

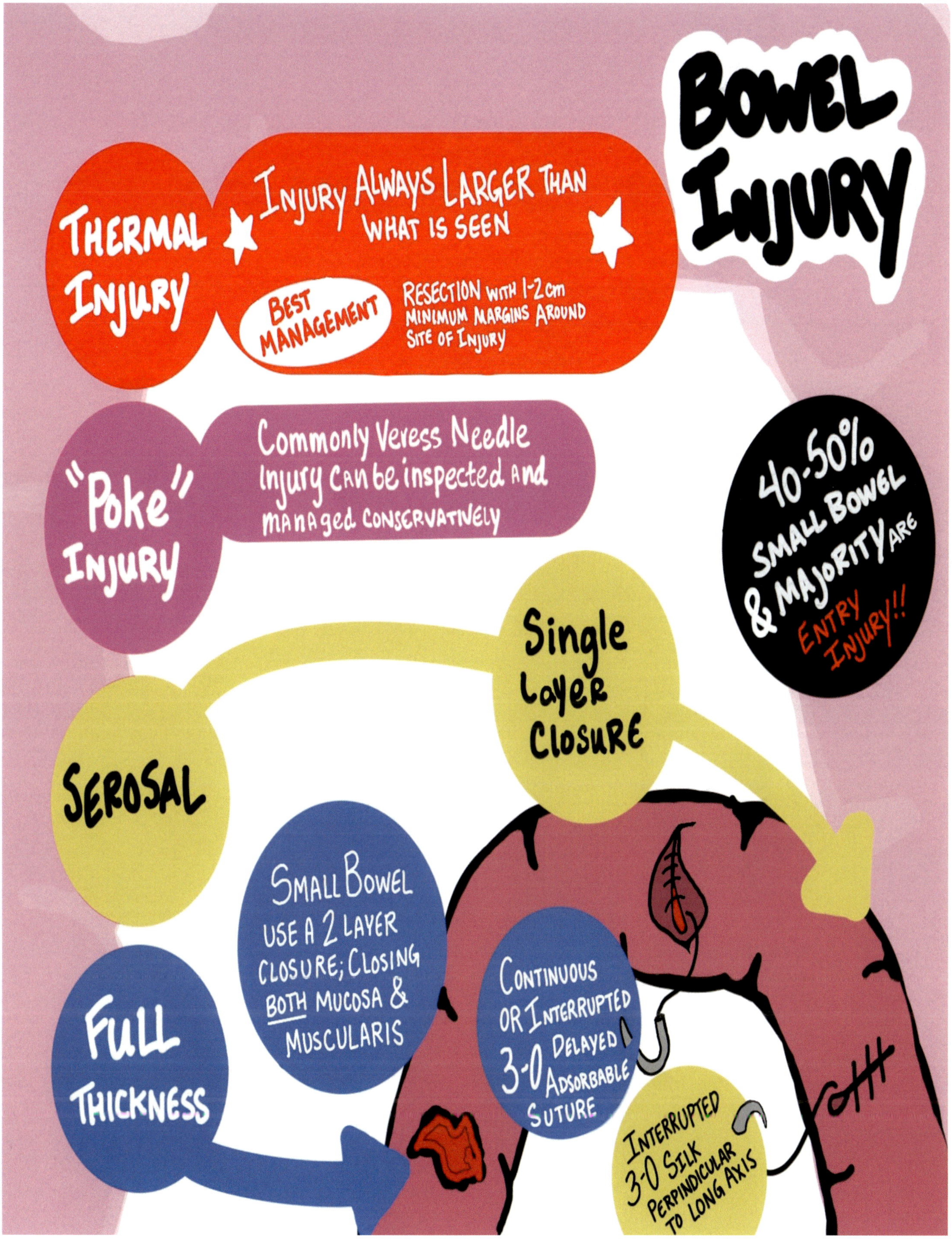
Bowel Injury
Thermal Injury
Injury Always Larger Than What is Seen
Best Management
Resection with 1-2cm minimum margins around site of injury
"Poke" Injury
Commonly Veress Needle Injury can be inspected and managed conservatively
40-50% Small Bowel & Majority are Entry Injury!!
Serosal
Single Layer Closure
Full Thickness
Small Bowel use a 2 layer closure; closing both mucosa & muscularis
Continuous or Interrupted 3-0 Delayed Adsorbable Suture
Interrupted 3-0 Silk Perpindicular to long axis

Blood Products and Administration

Being in a surgical speciality demands knowledge of blood products, their administration and when they are indicated. This drawing is a quick splattering of blood types and some of the screening that blood undergoes. You should also be aware of the risks of transmission of disease via blood products.

The image shows the derivation of blood products from whole blood. Give close attention to clotting factors, ABO and Rh requirements, volumes and what affect they have when given.

Some important OB/GYN High Yield Tips would be:

- Average (70 kg) female's blood volume is approximately 4000 mL
- Fetal blood volume varies by gestational age for calculation:
    - Preterm = 90 mL / kg (approximately 125 mL)
    - Term = 100 mL / kg (approximately 350 mL)
- Placenta at term averages = 125 - 150 mL of blood volume
- Fibrinogen is Factor 1 and Prothrombin is Factor 2

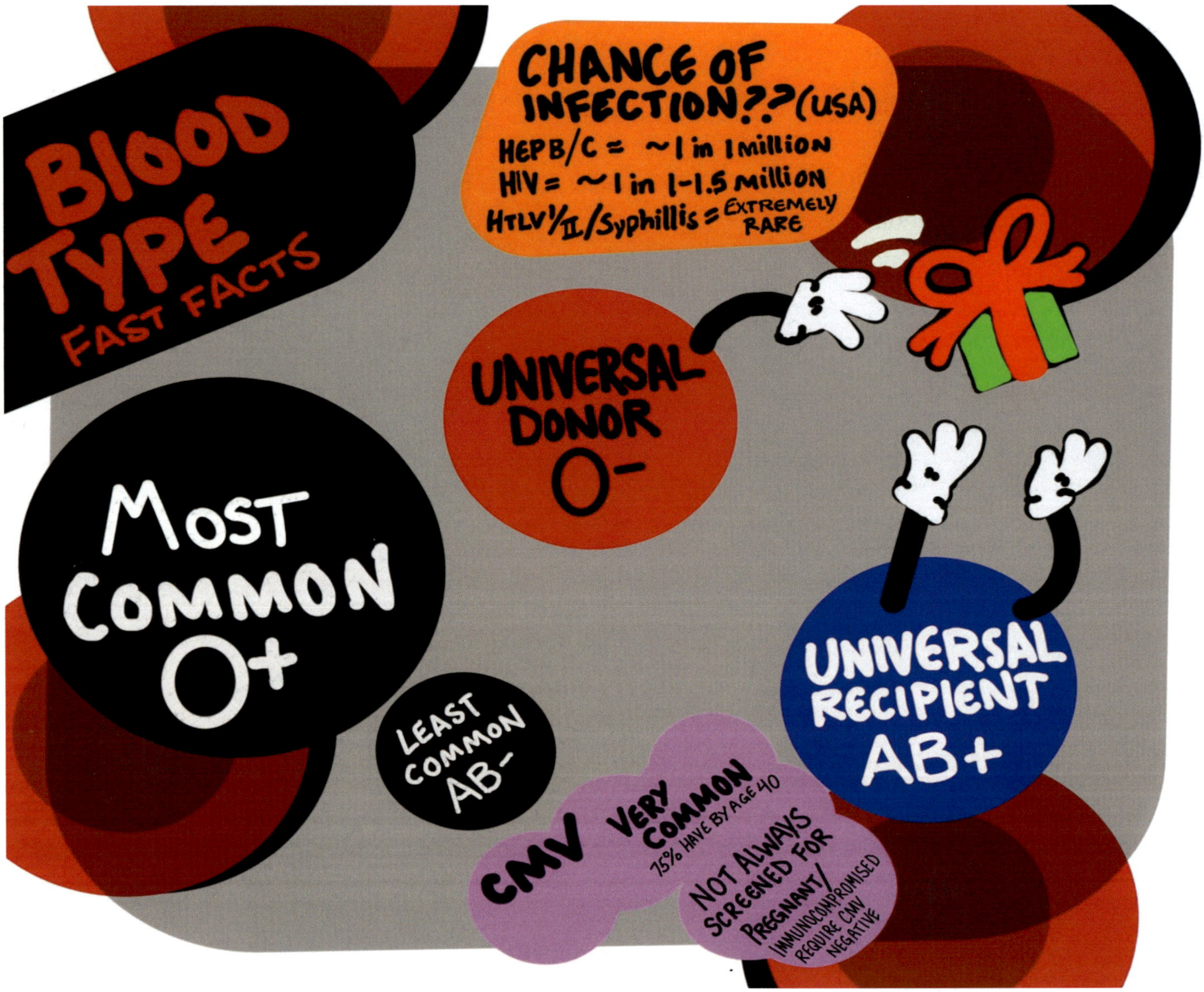
Blood Type
Fast Facts
Chance of Infection?? (USA)
HepB/C = ~1 in 1 million
HIV = ~1 in 1-1.5 million
HTLV I/II/Syphillis = Extremely rare
Universal Donor O-
Most Common O+
Least Common AB-
Universal Recipient AB+
CMV Very Common
75% have by age 40
Not always screened for
Pregnant/Immunocompromised require CMV negative

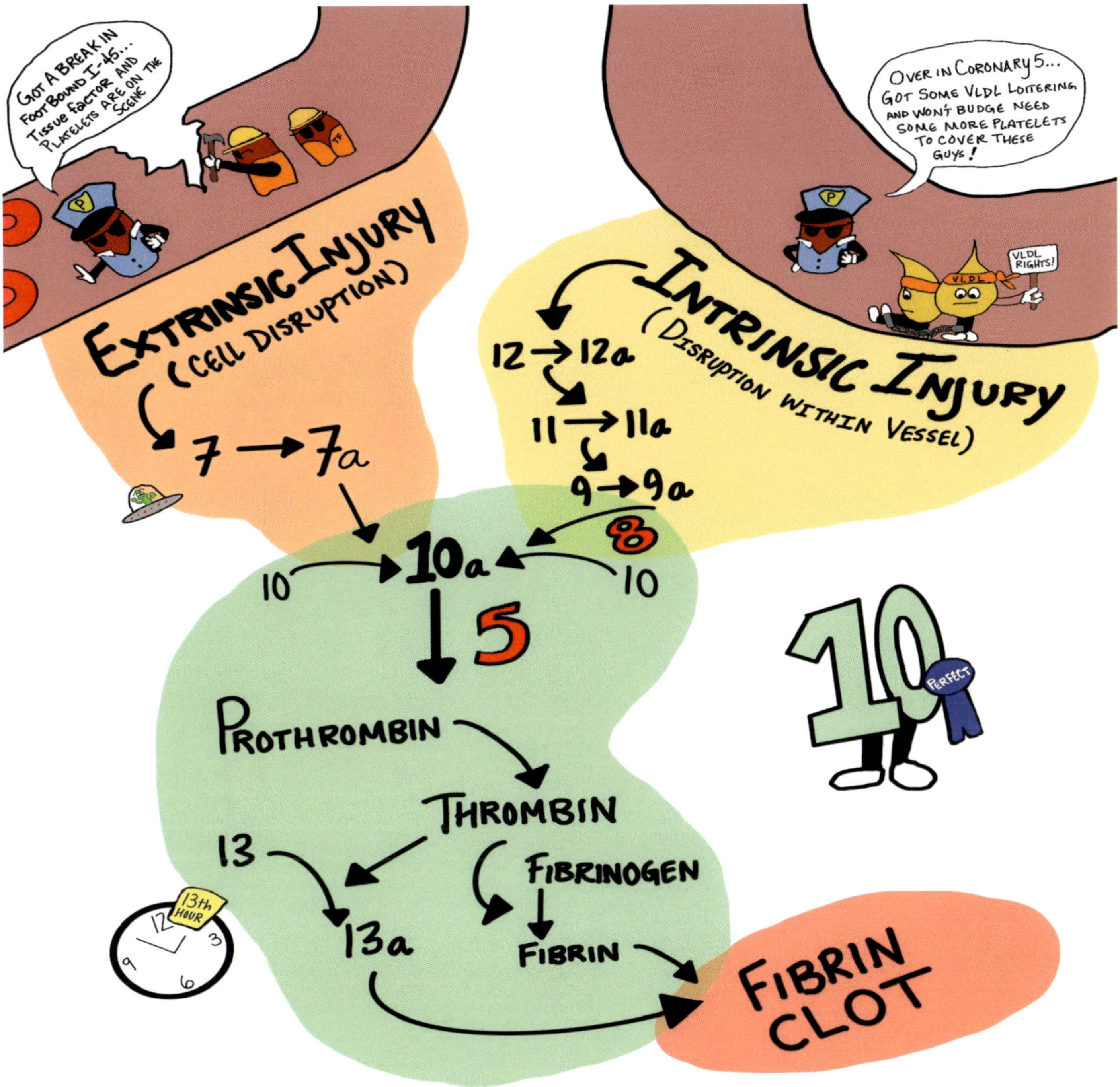

The Clotting Cascade

Special points of interest in the cascade include realizing the Extrinsic System is triggered by an injury that damages the vessel by disrupting the vascular wall. The Intrinsic system is the result of a disruption within the lumen of the vessel. The Extrinsic pathway has one unique factor; factor 7. Seven and the word Alien both have 5 letters and an alien visits Earth, which also has 5 letters, and he is all alone (5 letters look at that).

Think "perfect 10" to remind you that this is the factor that combines the two pathways making the common pathway.

The last factor to play a role in the "final hour" is 13. So, we think of the 13th hour.

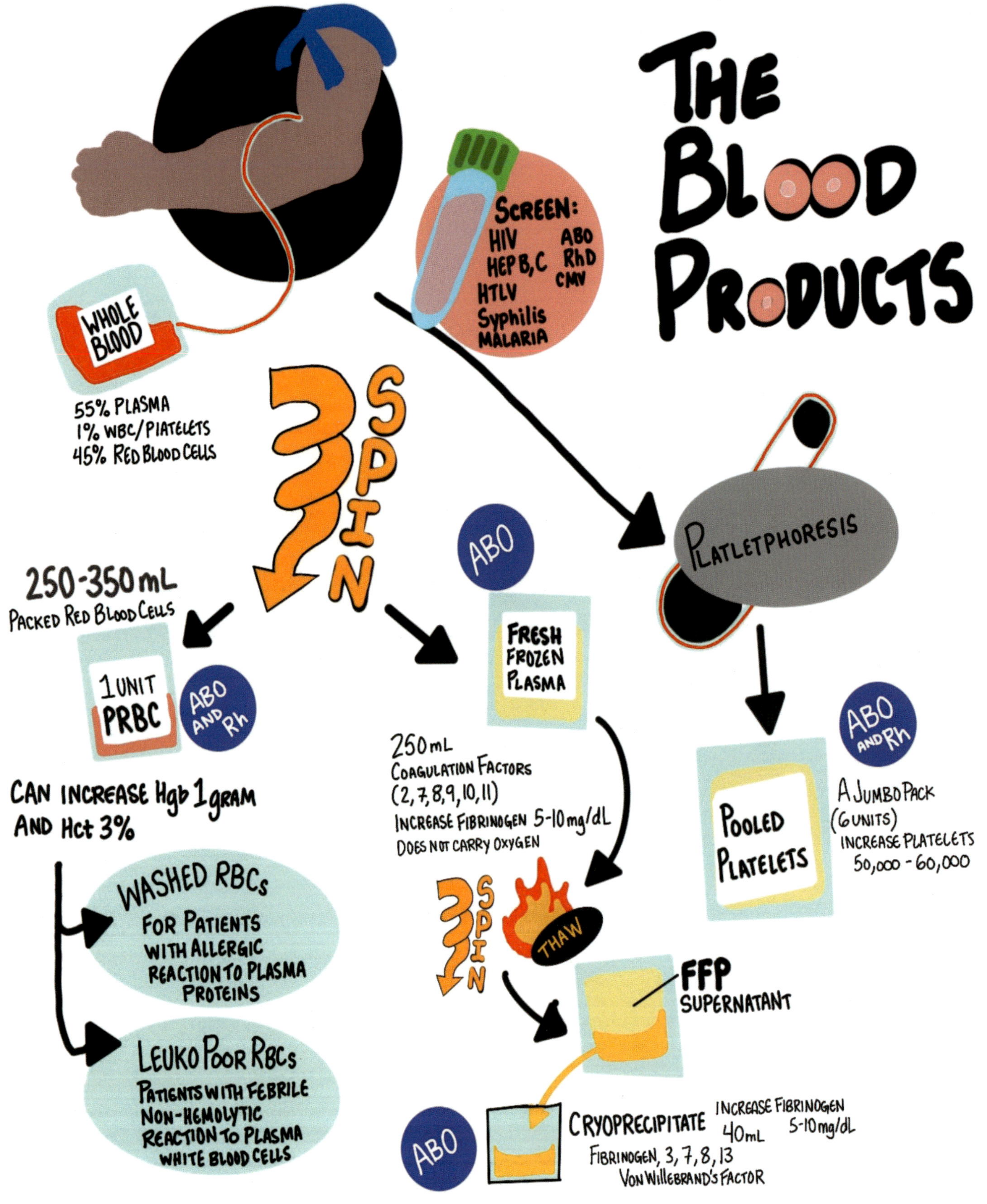
THE BLOOD PRODUCTS
SCREEN:
HIV
HEP B, C
HTLV
Syphilis
MALARIA
ABO
RhD
CMV
WHOLE BLOOD
55% PLASMA
1% WBC/PLATELETS
45% RED BLOOD CELLS
SPIN
250-350 mL
PACKED RED BLOOD CELLS
1 UNIT PRBC
ABO AND Rh
CAN INCREASE Hgb 1 GRAM AND Hct 3%
WASHED RBCs
FOR PATIENTS WITH ALLERGIC REACTION TO PLASMA PROTEINS
LEUKO POOR RBCs
PATIENTS WITH FEBRILE NON-HEMOLYTIC REACTION TO PLASMA WHITE BLOOD CELLS
ABO
FRESH FROZEN PLASMA
250 mL
COAGULATION FACTORS
(2, 7, 8, 9, 10, 11)
INCREASE FIBRINOGEN 5-10 mg/dL
DOES NOT CARRY OXYGEN
SPIN
THAW
FFP SUPERNATANT
ABO
CRYOPRECIPITATE
INCREASE FIBRINOGEN
40 mL
5-10 mg/dL
FIBRINOGEN, 3, 7, 8, 13
VON WILLEBRAND'S FACTOR
PLATLETPHORESIS
ABO AND Rh
POOLED PLATELETS
A JUMBO PACK
(6 UNITS)
INCREASE PLATELETS
50,000 - 60,000

Heparin and Low Molecular Weight Heparin

These will always be found on your exams and will either ask for the antidote or look for the understanding of their mechanisms. The drawing shows the "**IN**" in Hepar"**IN**" in orange and then this repeats in the words "**IN"**direct Thromb"**IN**" "**IN"**hibitor, which is to help you remember its unique mechanism of action. Also, Hepar"**IN**" also has affect on the "**IN"direct coagulation pathway.** Another tip for remembering the monitoring lab for Heparin are that the two T's in PTT can form a capital H, where just PT cannot.

Commonly seen questions have involved the following:

1. When should the medications be stopped preoperatively and when resumed?
2. Can a patient receive LMWH after Heparin Induced Thrombocytopenia?
3. What is the pathophysiology of Heparin Induced Thrombocytopenia?
4. When does Heparin therapy require bridging and does LMWH ever require this?

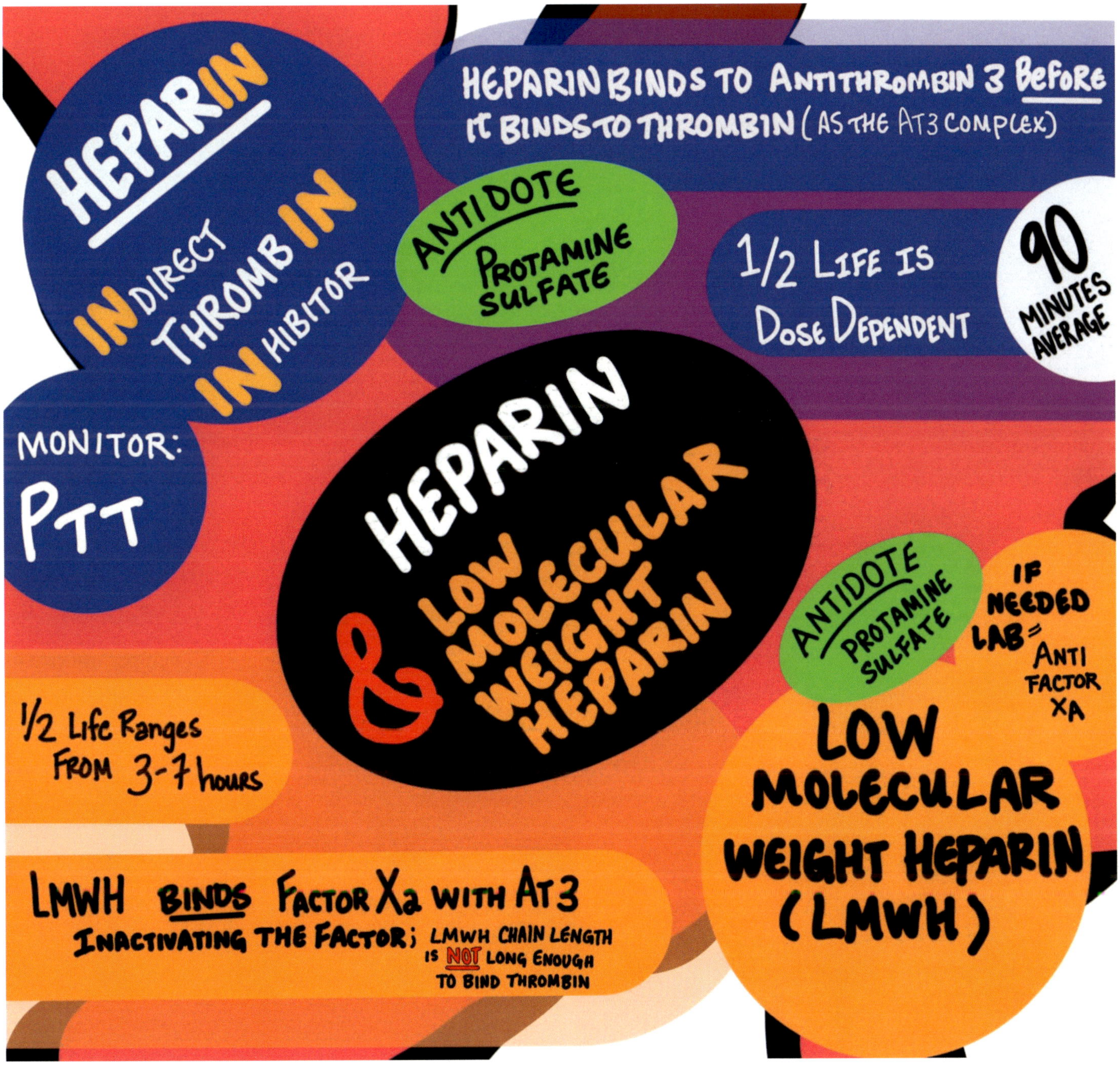
HEPARIN
INDIRECT THROMBIN INHIBITOR
HEPARIN BINDS TO ANTITHROMBIN 3 BEFORE IT BINDS TO THROMBIN (AS THE AT3 COMPLEX)
ANTIDOTE PROTAMINE SULFATE
1/2 LIFE IS DOSE DEPENDENT
90 MINUTES AVERAGE
MONITOR: PTT
HEPARIN & LOW MOLECULAR WEIGHT HEPARIN
ANTIDOTE PROTAMINE SULFATE
IF NEEDED LAB = ANTI FACTOR XA
1/2 Life Ranges FROM 3-7 hours
LOW MOLECULAR WEIGHT HEPARIN (LMWH)
LMWH BINDS FACTOR Xa WITH AT3 INACTIVATING THE FACTOR; LMWH CHAIN LENGTH IS NOT LONG ENOUGH TO BIND THROMBIN

Wound Classification and Antibiotics

In every operating room during time-out you will be asked if your patient needs antibiotics for the procedure/ surgery. It is essential that you understand wound classification and when antibiotics are necessary. These questions are classics on the board examinations and it usually starts as one type and changes due to enterotomy or other surgical complication. Remember for oral boards, if your wound class changes and the new class requires antibiotics, you need to say it!

The birds will help you remember which classes need antibiotics (Green birds = Yes). A good rule of thumb for antibiotics is…if you don't make contact between the intraperitoneal space and the vagina/lining of the endometrium (including backfilling the uterus and spilling into the peritoneum), then you usually don't need antibiotics.

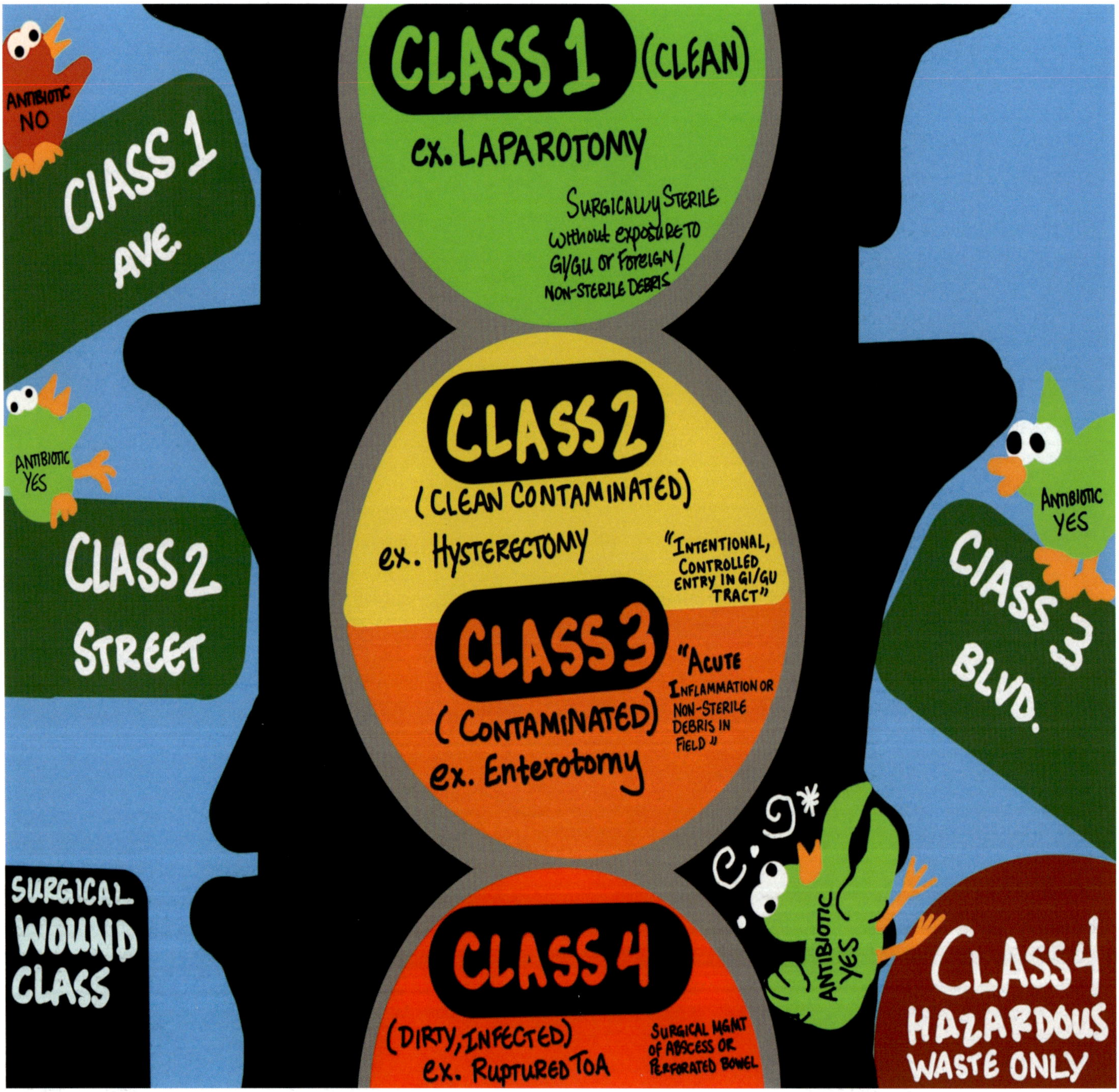

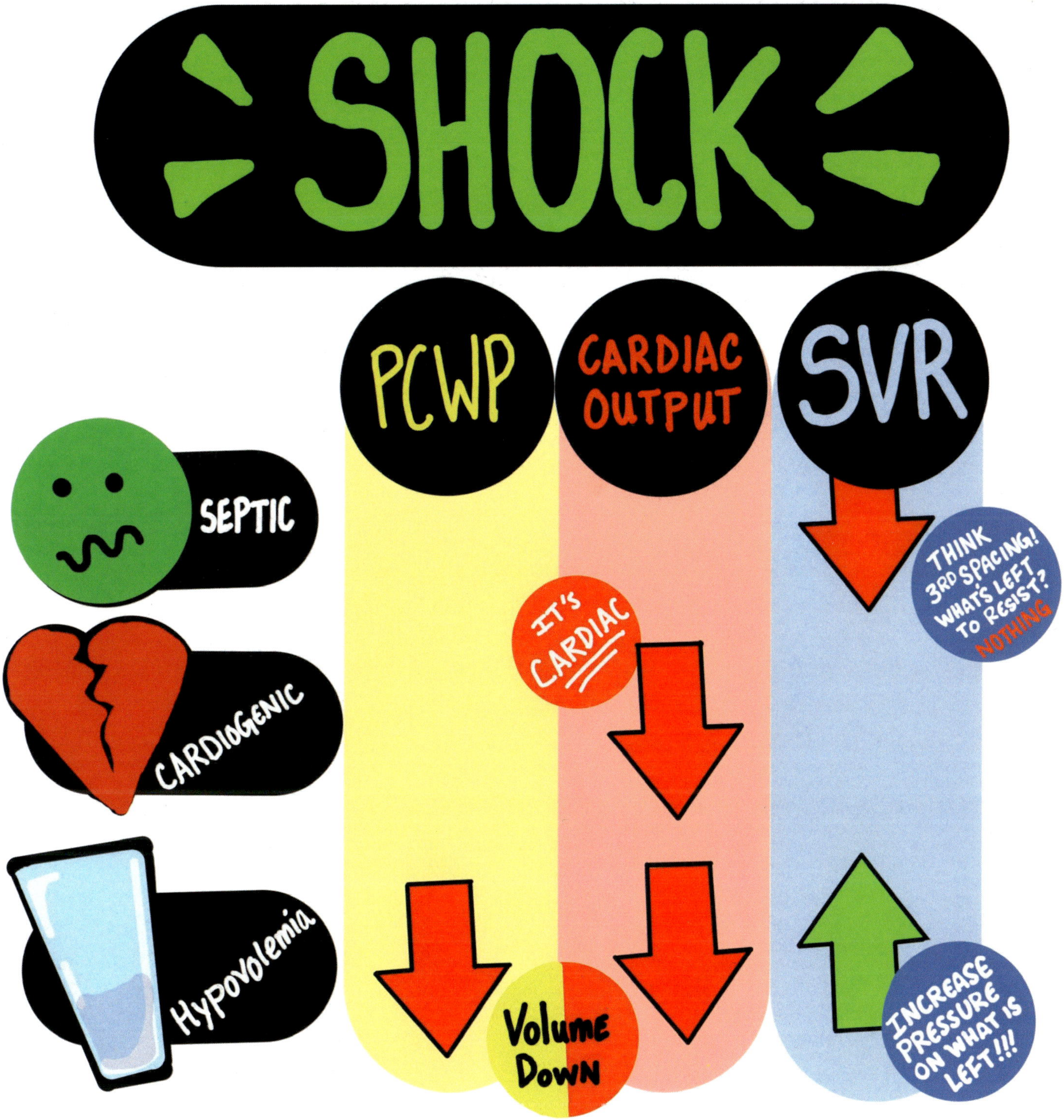

Shock

This is a topic that has been known to sneak into the exam. You don't want to miss a question because you don't remember the affects of Shock on Pulmonary Capillary Wedge Pressure (PCWP) or how the Cardiac Output changes. Most importantly, make sure you make sense of Systemic Vascular Resistance (SVR) as this can be the measurement that differentiates one clinical picture from another.

Also, Hypovolemic and Cardiogenic shock have been favorite Obstetric questions in the past.

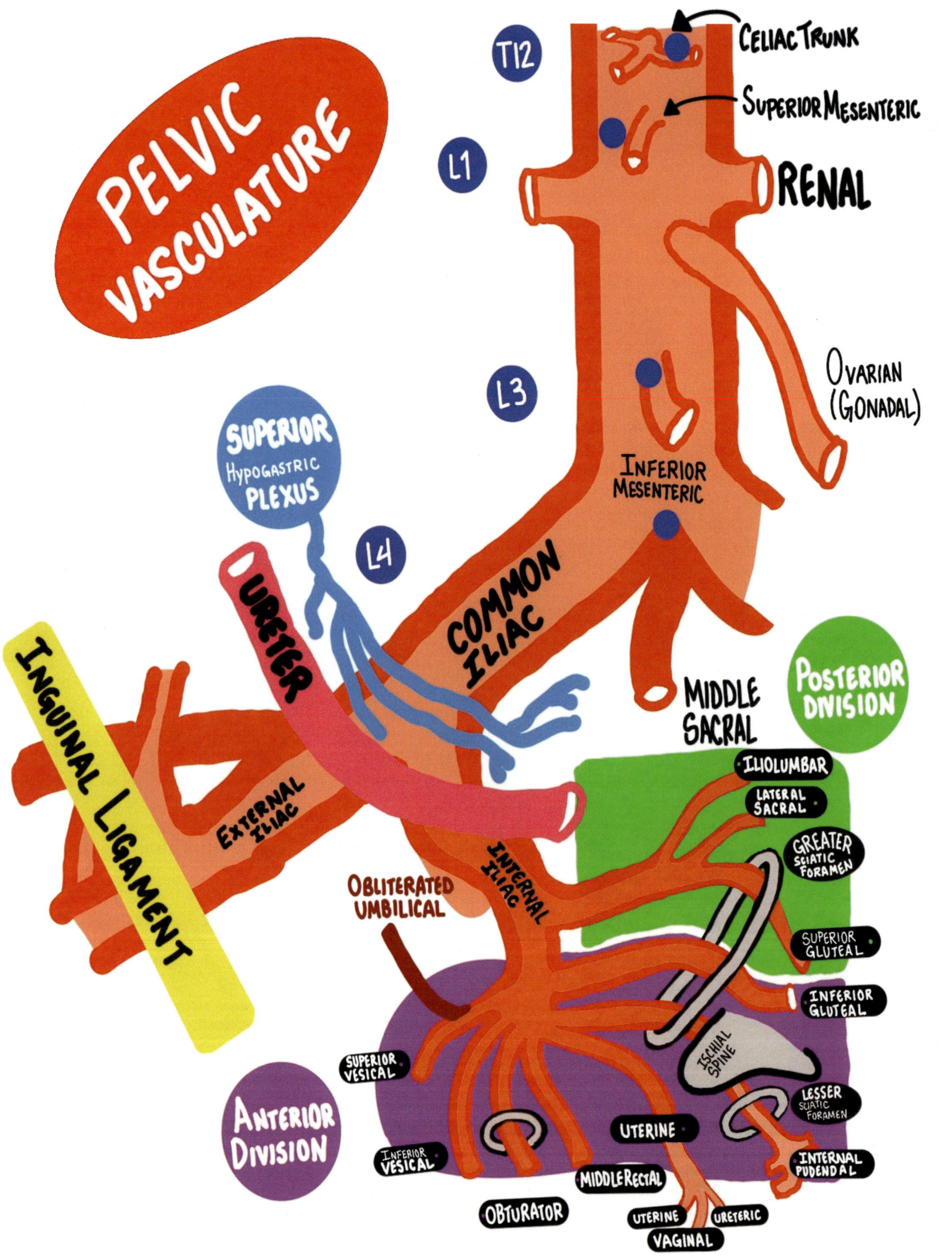
PELVIC VASCULATURE
T12
CELIAC TRUNK
SUPERIOR MESENTERIC
L1
RENAL
OVARIAN (GONADAL)
L3
INFERIOR MESENTERIC
SUPERIOR Hypogastric PLEXUS
L4
URETER
COMMON ILIAC
INGUINAL LIGAMENT
EXTERNAL ILIAC
MIDDLE SACRAL
POSTERIOR DIVISION
ILIOLUMBAR
LATERAL SACRAL
GREATER SCIATIC FORAMEN
INTERNAL ILIAC
OBLITERATED UMBILICAL
SUPERIOR GLUTEAL
INFERIOR GLUTEAL
ISCHIAL SPINE
SUPERIOR VESICAL
LESSER SCIATIC FORAMEN
ANTERIOR DIVISION
UTERINE
INFERIOR VESICAL
INTERNAL PUDENDAL
MIDDLE RECTAL
OBTURATOR
UTERINE
URETERIC
VAGINAL

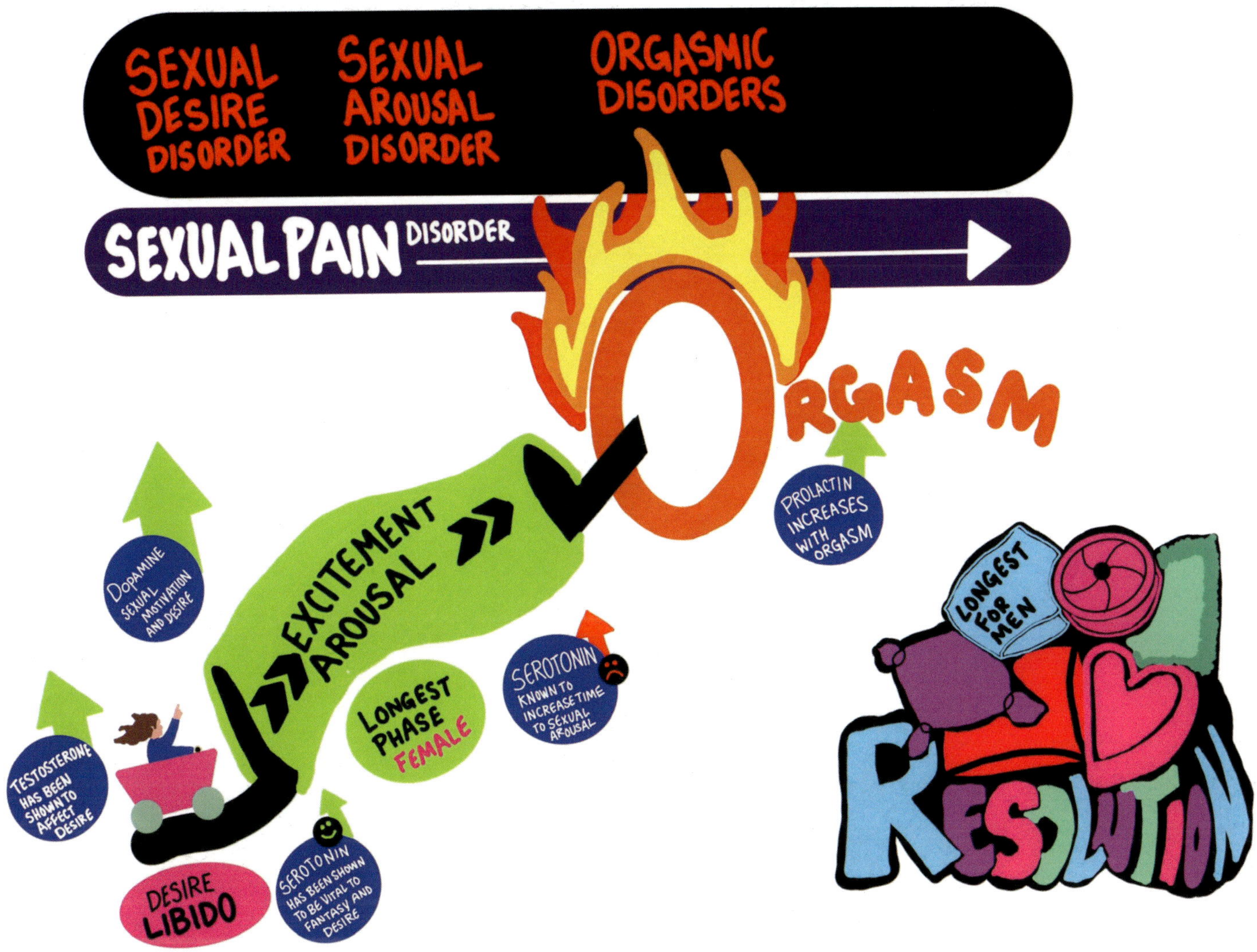

Sexual Dysfunction Disorders

Sexual Aversion Disorder - persistent or recurrent phobic avoidance of sexual contact

Non-coital Sexual Pain - genital pain following stimulation during foreplay

SSRI Medications - most likely cause of Orgasmic, Desire and Arousal Disorders

PHASE	DISORDER	NOTES	SOME TREATMENTS
Desire	Hypoactive Sexual Desire Disorder	Most Common Disorder	Transdermal Testosterone Phentolamine (Vasofem) Sidenafil (Viagra)
Excitement	Sexual Arousal Diorder, Dyspareunia, Vaginismus	Longest FEMALE Phase	Alprostadil/PGE_1 (Femprox, Alista) Vaginismis/Dyspareunia (Estrogen)
Orgasm	Orgasmic Disorder	Female Response Varies	
Resolution	Post Coital Dysphoria/ Headache	Female Response Varies, Longest MALE Phase	

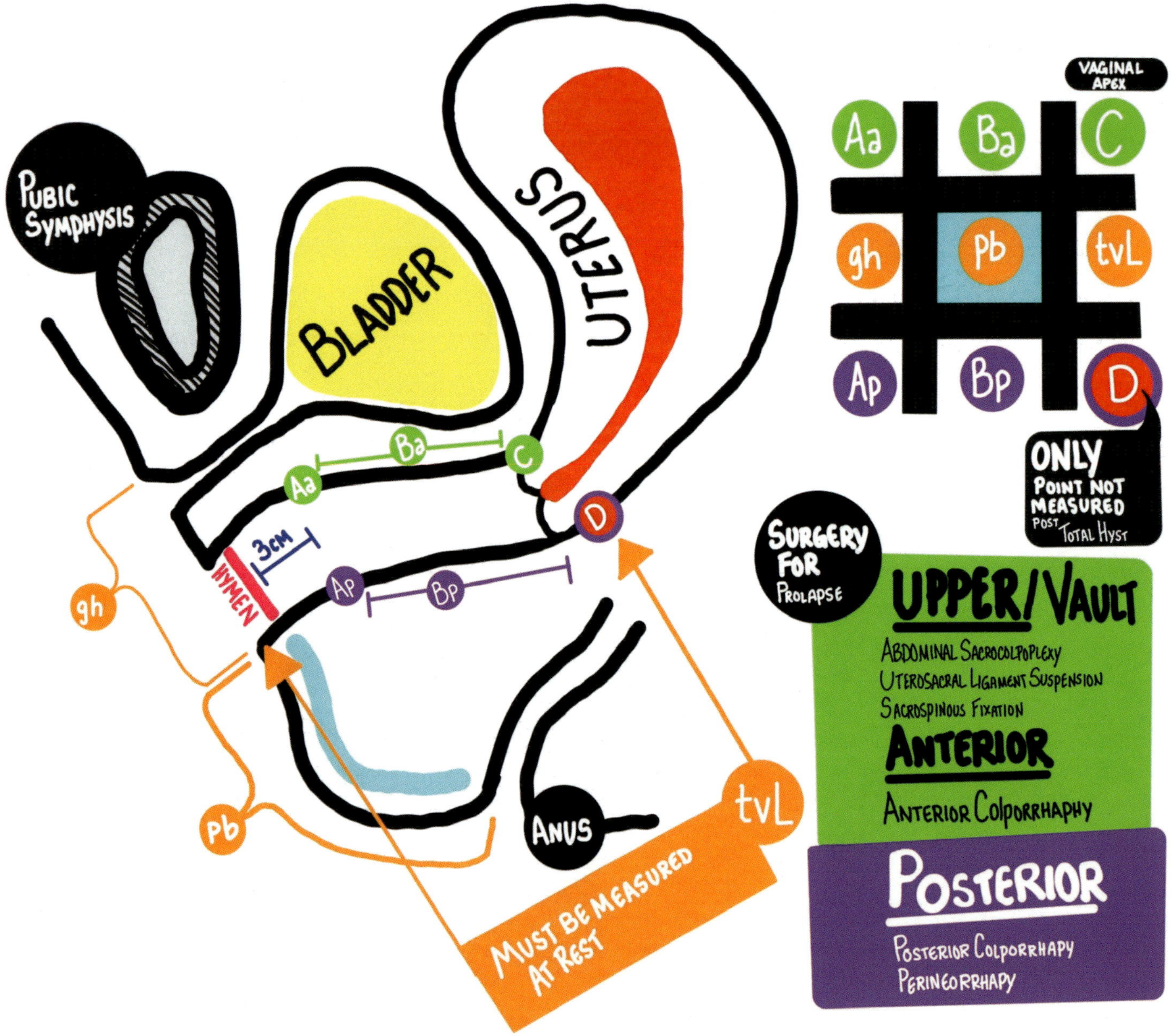

Pelvic Organ Prolapse

The most commonly asked questions surrounding this subject will be a POP-Q score or a description of a prolapse in terms of measurements and presentation. You should be familiar with how the system works and how the measurements are made.

Some of the important things to remember:

-Total Vaginal Length must be measured in an independent or "at rest" position

-Point D is NOT PRESENT after a TOTAL hysterectomy

-gh has the least variability in measurement between providers

The next drawing will explain the staging of pelvic organ prolapse.

Pelvic Organ Prolapse

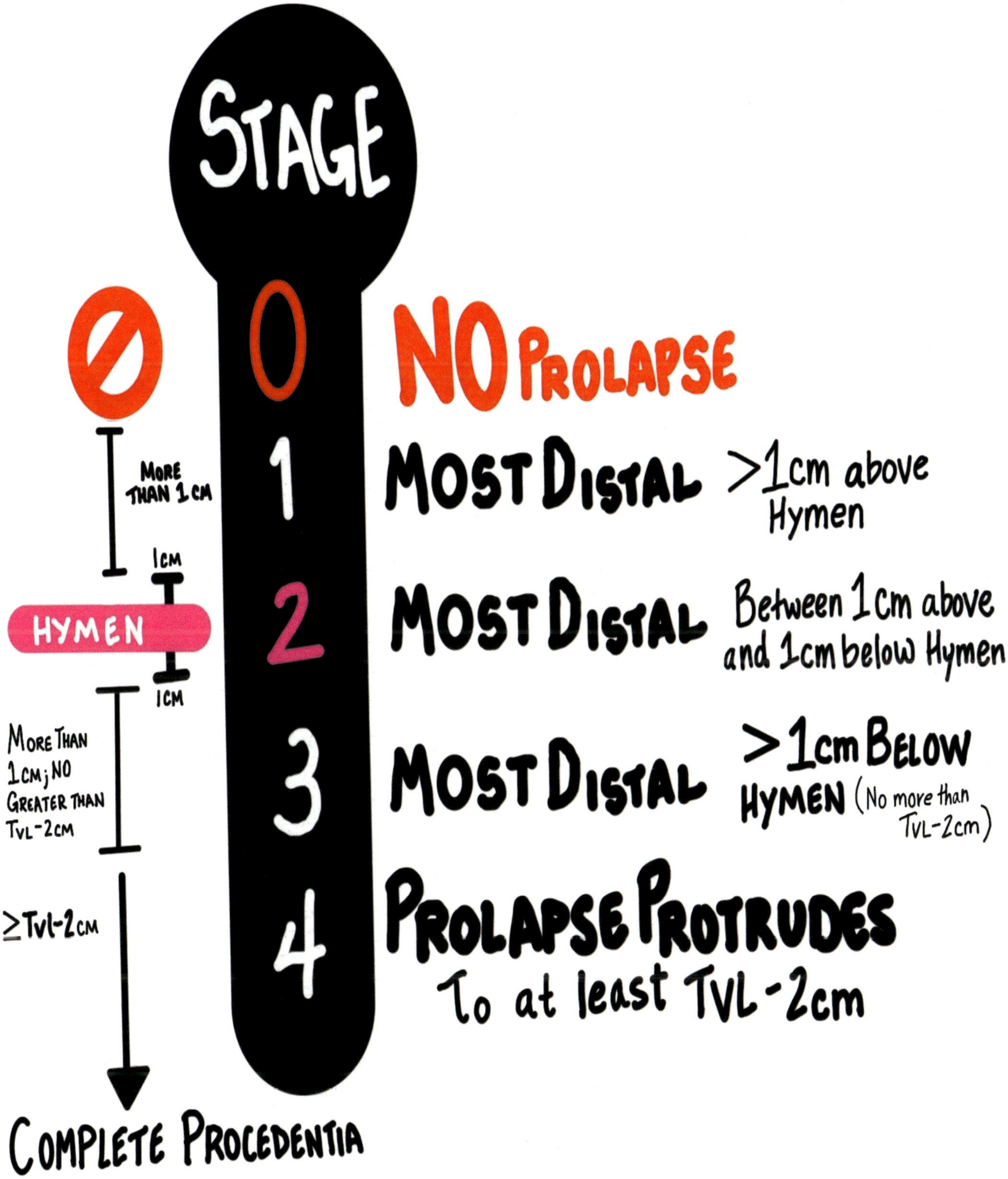

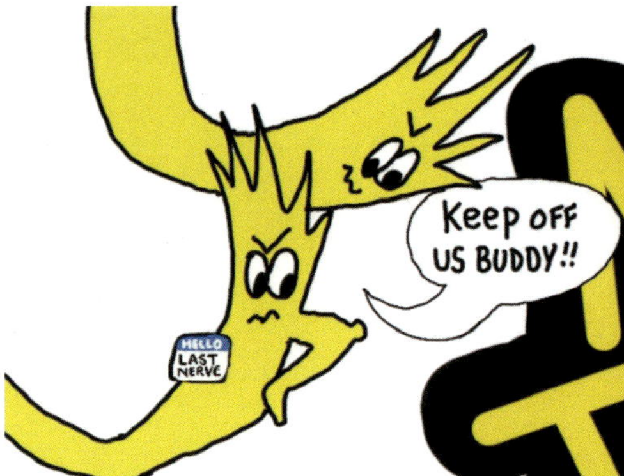

NERVE INJURY

FREQUENCY	SIGNS/SYMPTOMS	NERVE
20-30%	Numbness anteromedial thigh, Weak external rotation, Weak adduction	Obturator L2-4
11-30%	Numbness anteromedial thigh, Weak leg extension, Weak flexion of hip, Absent knee jerk	Femoral L2-4
17%	Numbness/burning pain upper labia and thigh (Sensory only)	Genitofemoral L1-2
10%	Numbness foot/leg, Foot drop, Buttock pain, posterior/lateral leg pain	Lumbosacral/ sciatic L4-S3
7%	Sharp/cutting pain usually delayed pain lower abdomen (Sensory only)	Illioinguinal/ Iliohypogastric T12-L1
6%	Numbness, lateral thigh or hyperesthesia	Lateral Femoral Cutaneous

Peroneal Nerve
4 Fs: Fibular head
Foot drop
4 Nerve root (L3-S2)
Fin (yellow fin for lithotomy stirrups)

GYNECOLOGICAL ONCOLOGY

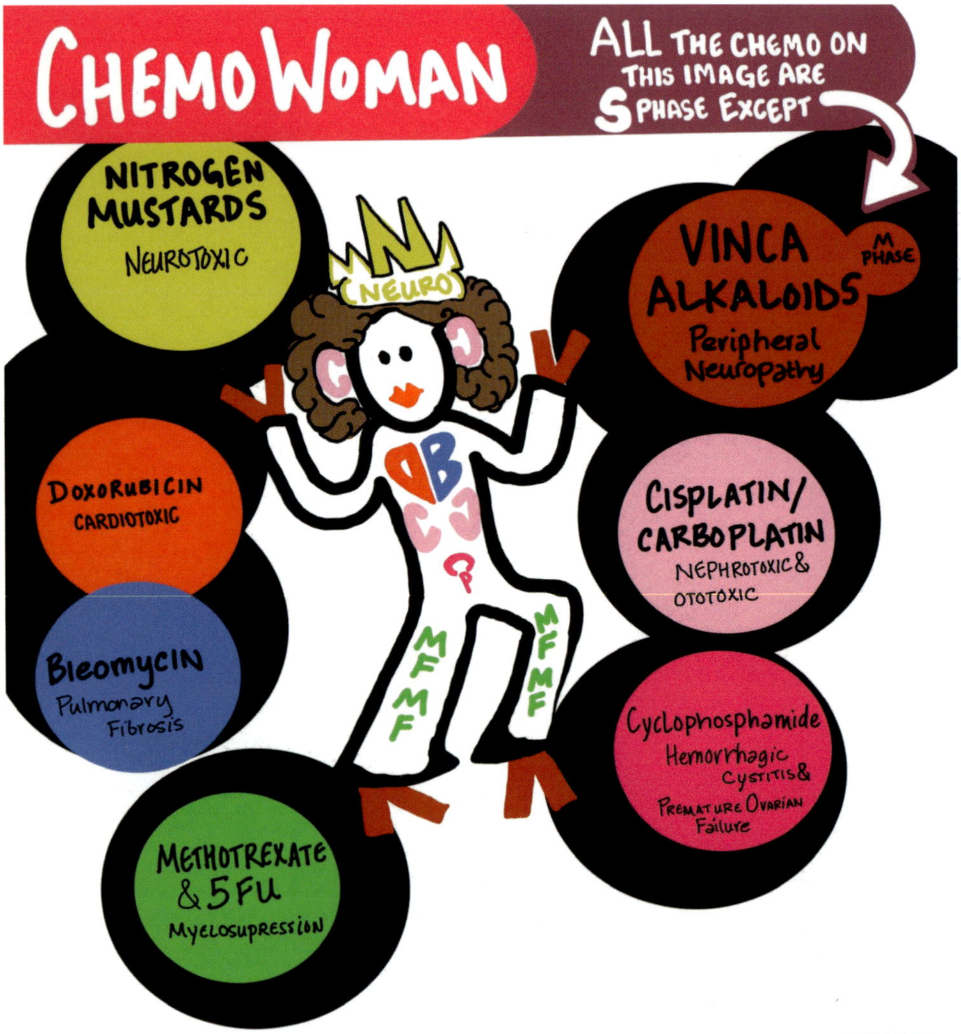

CHEMO WOMAN
ALL THE CHEMO ON THIS IMAGE ARE S PHASE EXCEPT
NITROGEN MUSTARDS
NEUROTOXIC
NEURO
VINCA ALKALOIDS
M PHASE
Peripheral Neuropathy
DOXORUBICIN
CARDIOTOXIC
OB
CISPLATIN/ CARBOPLATIN
NEPHROTOXIC & OTOTOXIC
Bleomycin
Pulmonary Fibrosis
MFMF
MFMF
Cyclophosphamide
Hemorrhagic cystitis & Premature Ovarian Failure
METHOTREXATE & 5FU
MYELOSUPRESSION

Chemotherapy and Adverse Effects

There will be many questions during your Gynecology Oncology portions of the exam on chemotherapy. Most common are the adverse and side effects of these agents. The others are usually related to their uses and how they work.

The Chemo Woman drawing is to help you quickly remember the main areas the "S" phase chemo agents effect. These are the most commonly asked.

Vinca Alkaloids are also on the chart. However, they are "M" phase agents.

The Cell Cycle drawing is a quick guide to where the different agents affect the cancer cells. You will definitely need to know these well.

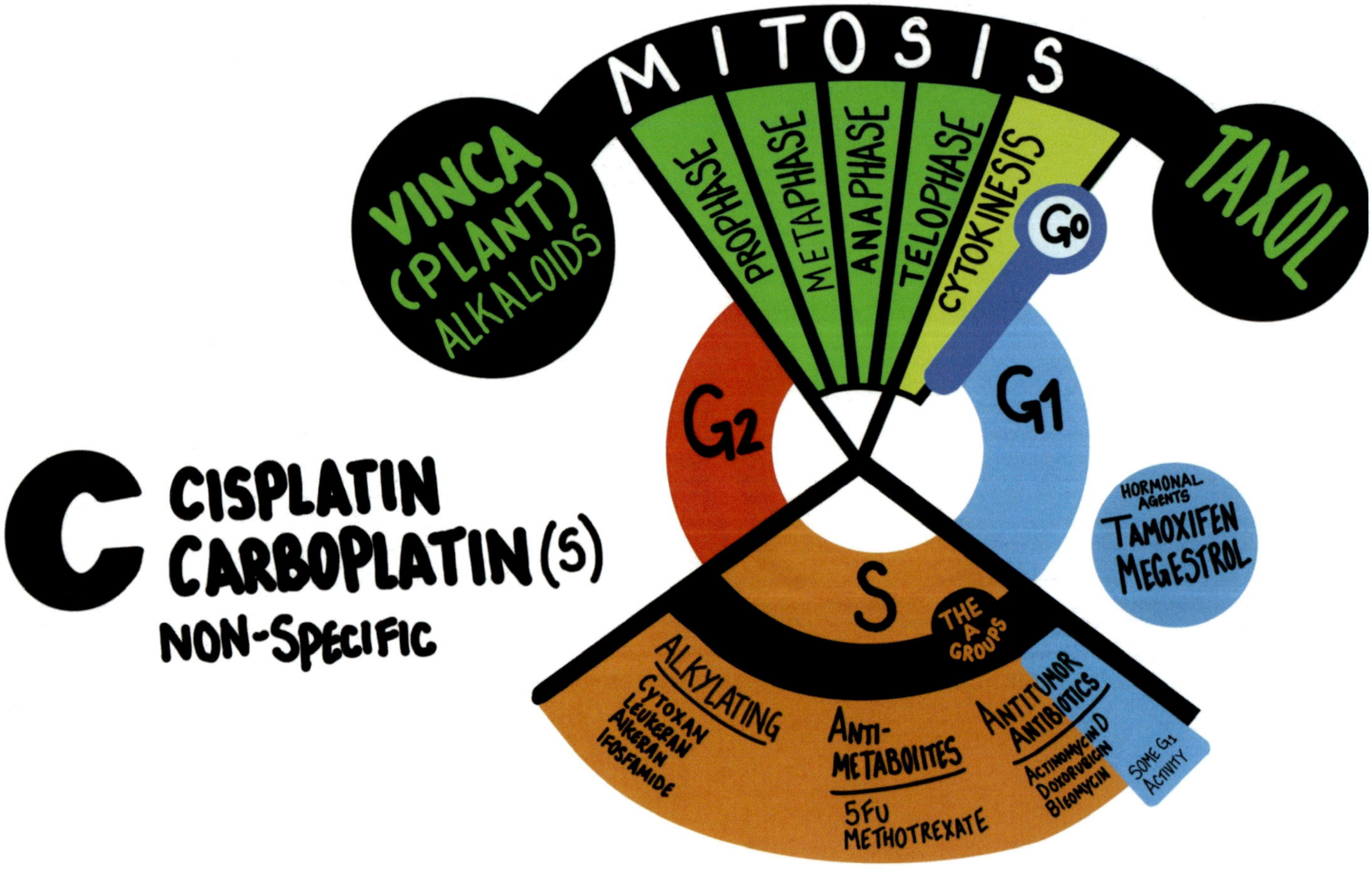

Ovarian Cancer

As we all know, Ovarian Cancer is a serious topic! Since it is an area of research for screening and testing to help diagnose the pathology earlier, it will be a common source of questions on your exams. According to the American Cancer Society, and agreed upon in the ACOG literature, the overall lifetime risk for any woman is about 1 in 78 - that's not rare! Subsequently, her lifetime risk of dying from that ovarian cancer is 1 in 108.

The drawing shows the risk for Epithelial versus Germ Cell in the different age groups of women. We also see the most common subtypes that are listed under each age group. The next drawings show the types and staging of ovarian cancer.

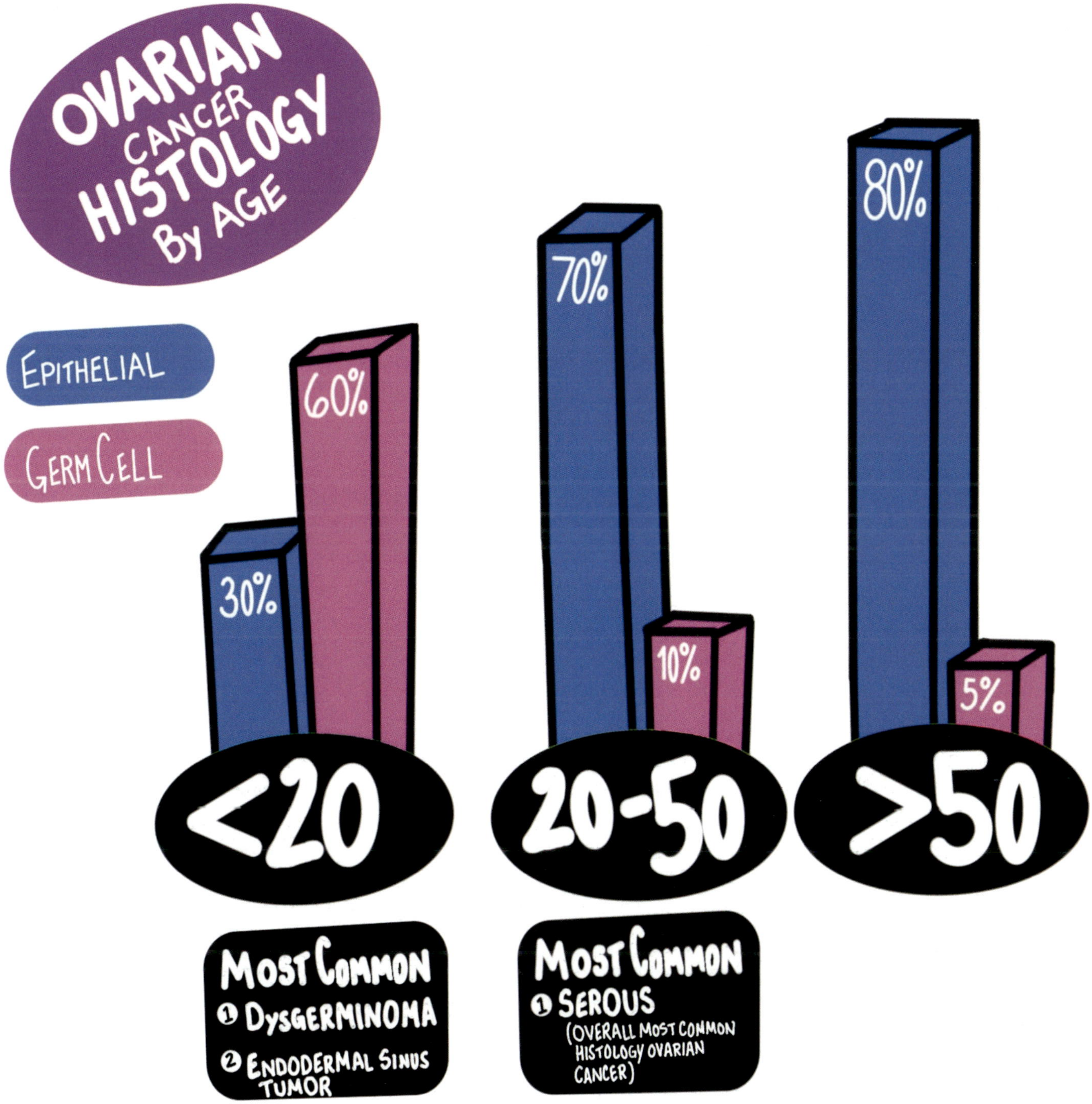

Ovarian Cancer Staging

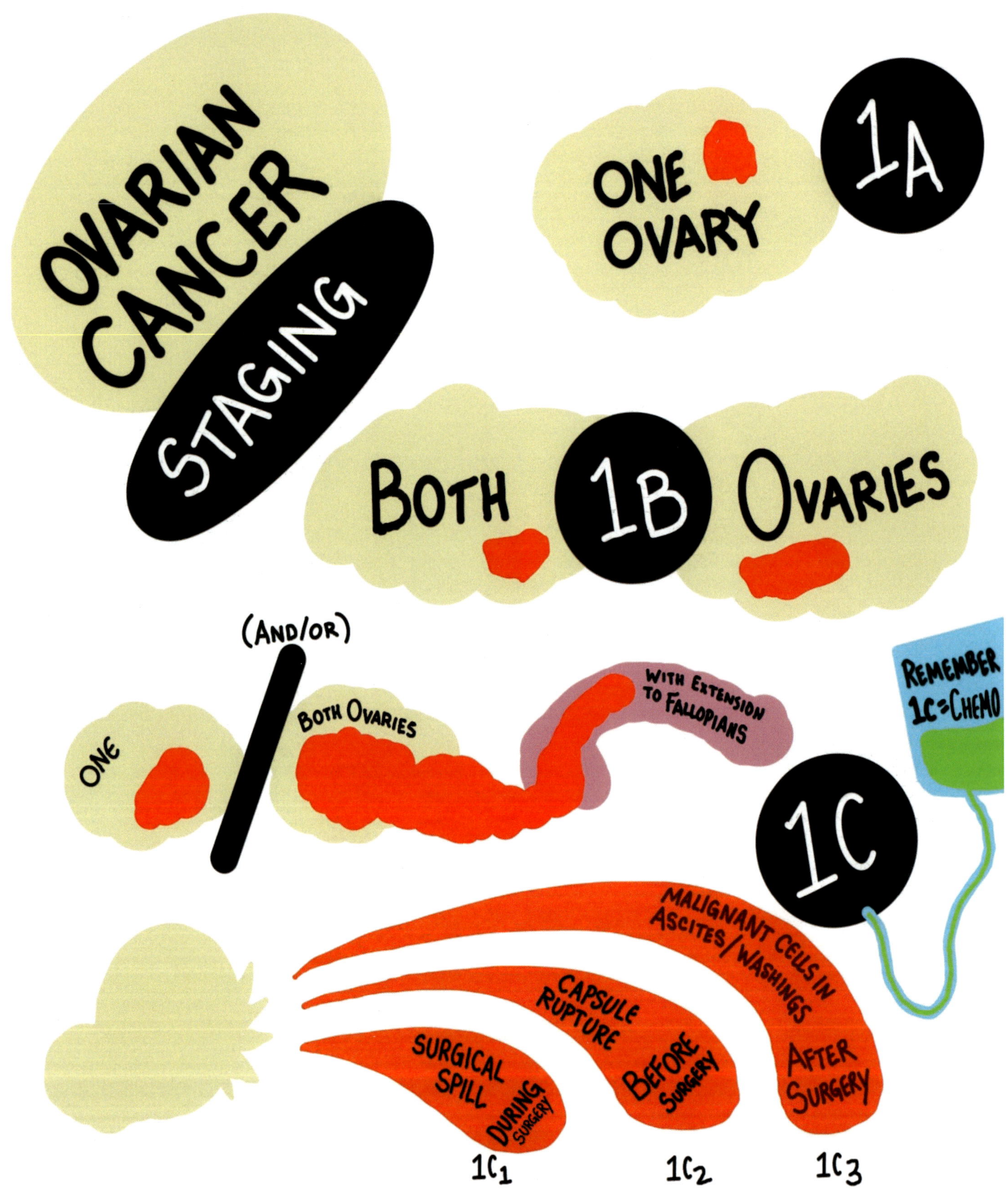

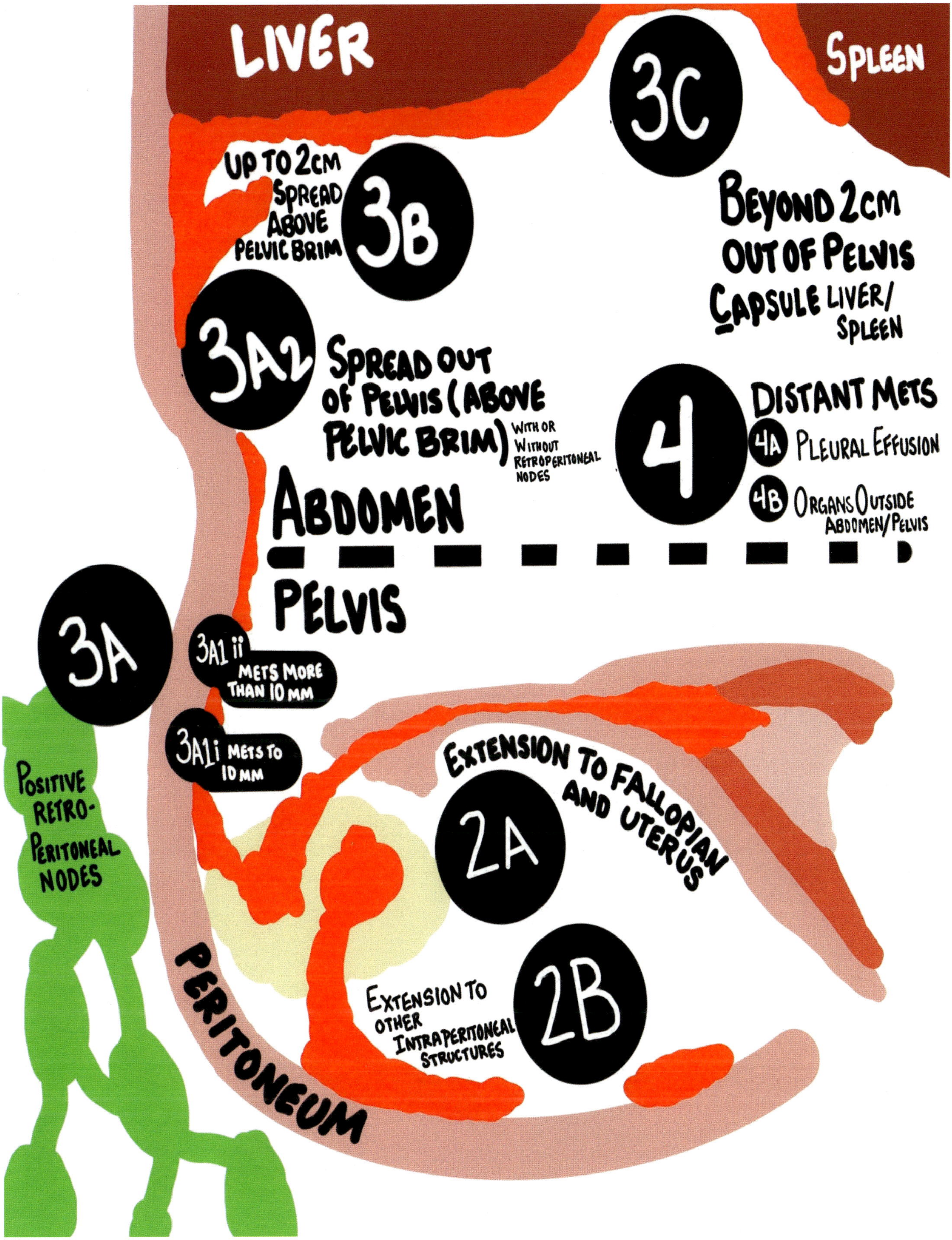
LIVER
SPLEEN
3C
UP TO 2CM SPREAD ABOVE PELVIC BRIM
3B
BEYOND 2CM OUT OF PELVIS
CAPSULE LIVER/SPLEEN
3A2
SPREAD OUT OF PELVIS (ABOVE PELVIC BRIM)
WITH OR WITHOUT RETROPERITONEAL NODES
4
DISTANT METS
4A PLEURAL EFFUSION
4B ORGANS OUTSIDE ABDOMEN/PELVIS
ABDOMEN
PELVIS
3A
3A1 ii METS MORE THAN 10 MM
3A1i METS TO 10 MM
POSITIVE RETRO-PERITONEAL NODES
EXTENSION TO FALLOPIAN AND UTERUS
2A
EXTENSION TO OTHER INTRAPERITONEAL STRUCTURES
2B
PERITONEUM

Ovarian Cancer Histology

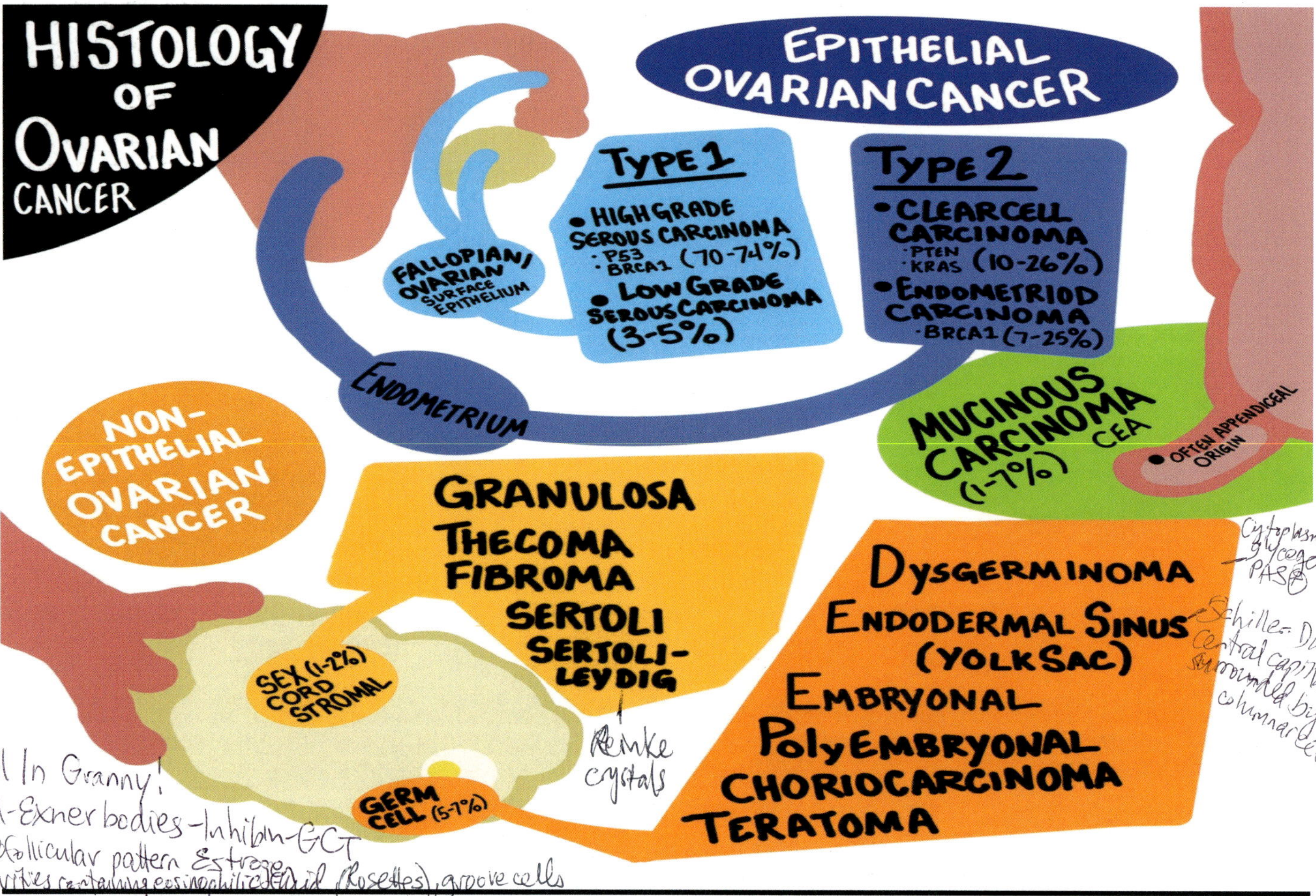

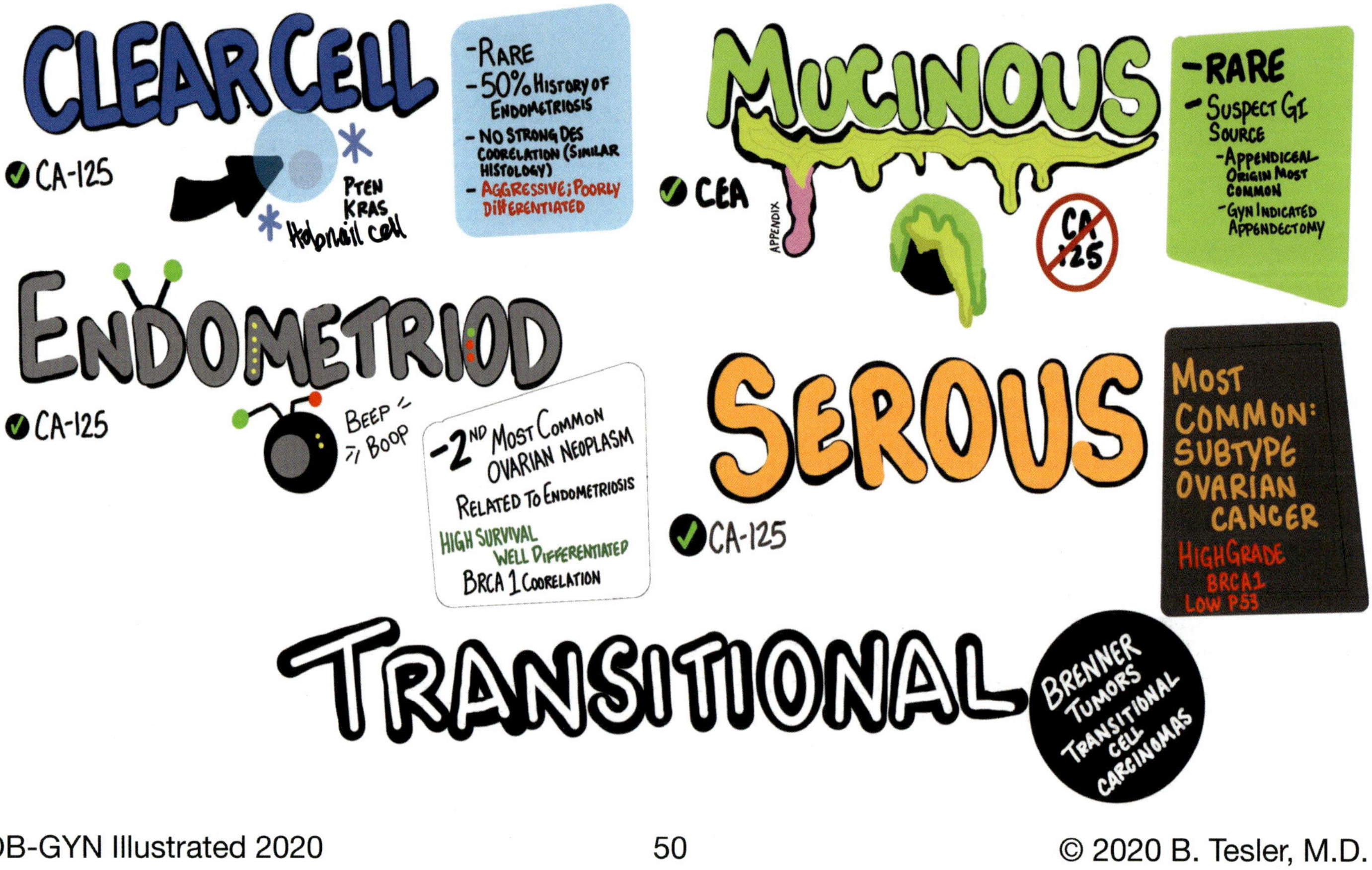

ENDOMETRIAL CANCER STAGING

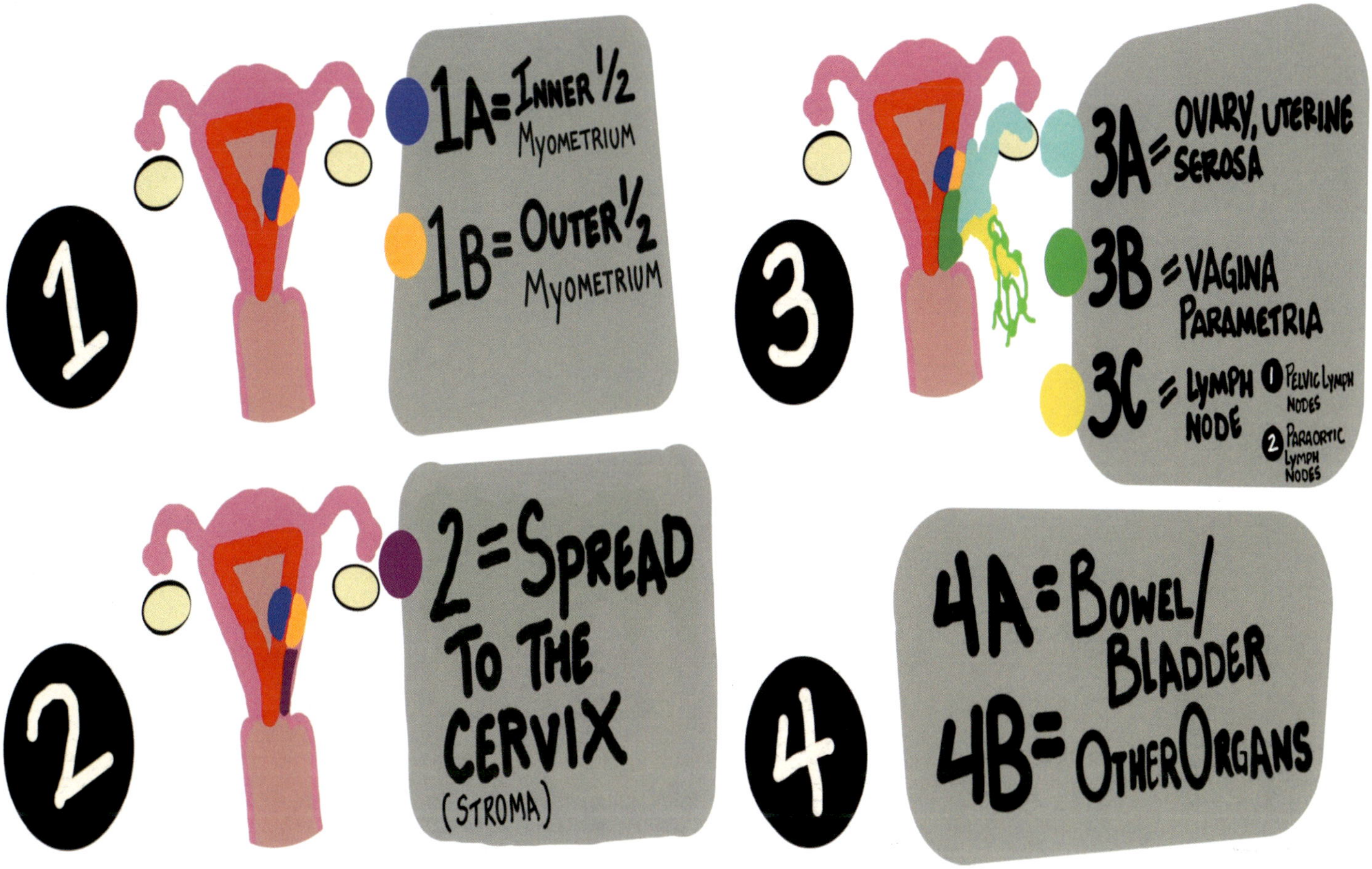

Endometrial Cancer

Endometrial Cancer is important to know for your exams because it is the MOST COMMON cancer of the female reproductive organs. This cancer usually affects postmenopausal women and the average age of diagnosis is about 60 years of age. The peak age distribution is 55 - 64 years of age. A woman's lifetime risk is about 1 in 39 for this type of cancer.

White women are more likely to develop Endometrial Cancer in their lifetimes than women of other races. However, Black women who develop endometrial cancer are more likely to die from the cancer.

The risk factors of Endometrial Cancer include from the most to least:

- Unopposed Estrogen Therapy
- Estrogen Producing Tumors
- Tamoxifen Usage
- Obesity
- Nulliparity/Infertility
- Diabetes Mellitus
- Menstrual Factors

Protective factors for Endometrial Cancer are: Cigarette Smoking, Combined Oral Contraceptive Use

Uterine Cancer

Technically, this category includes both Mensenchymal Sarcoma Subtypes (3%) and Endometrial Carcinoma (97%). However, we have already covered Endometrial Cancer. Therefore, as a total group, Uterine Cancer is the 4th most common female cancer in the United States and the MOST COMMON (due to endometrial) female reproductive tract cancer.

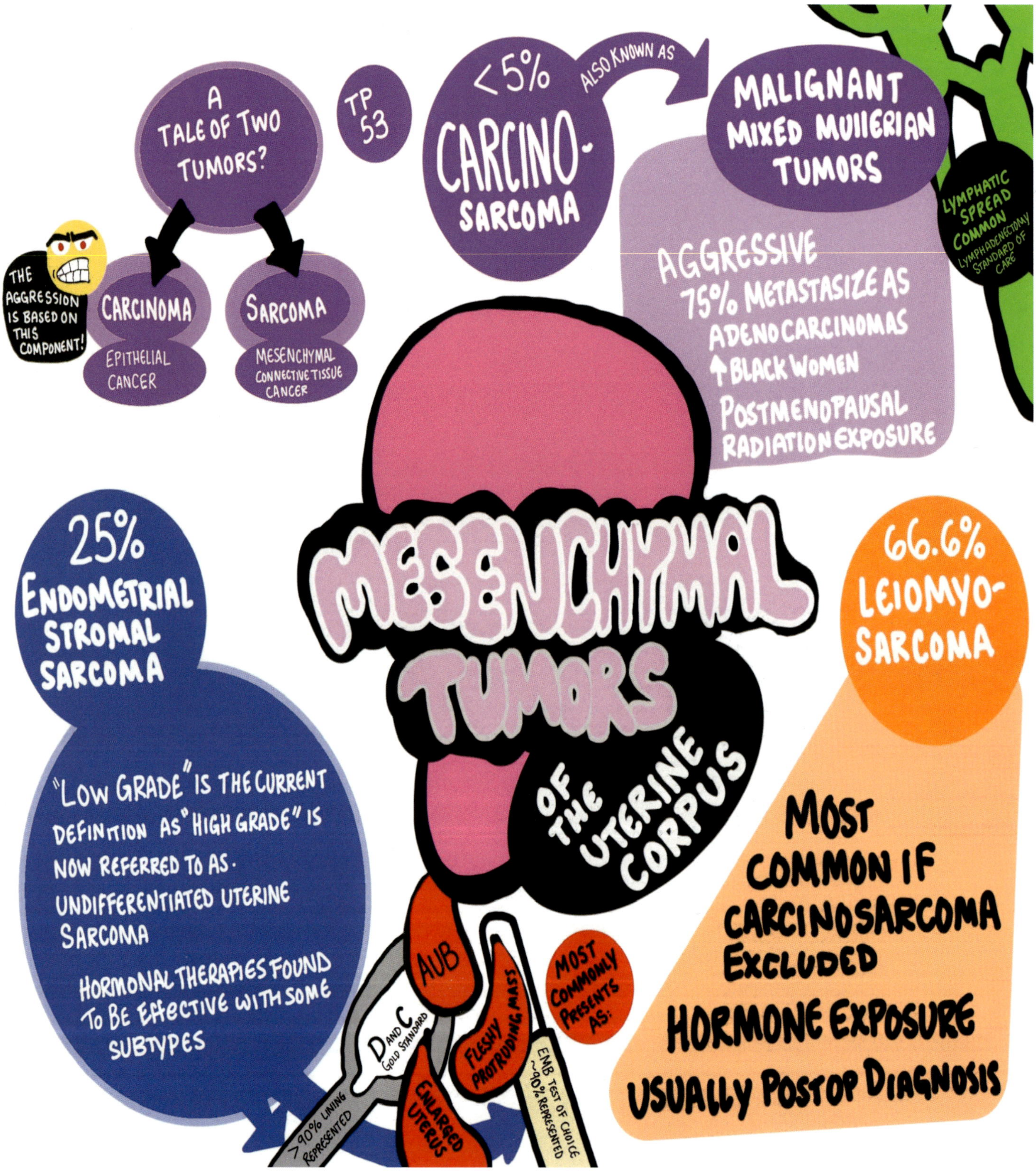

A TALE OF TWO TUMORS?
CARCINOMA
EPITHELIAL CANCER
SARCOMA
MESENCHYMAL CONNECTIVE TISSUE CANCER
THE AGGRESSION IS BASED ON THIS COMPONENT!
TP 53
<5% CARCINO-SARCOMA
ALSO KNOWN AS
MALIGNANT MIXED MULLERIAN TUMORS
AGGRESSIVE
75% METASTASIZE AS ADENOCARCINOMAS
↑ BLACK WOMEN
POSTMENOPAUSAL
RADIATION EXPOSURE
LYMPHATIC SPREAD COMMON
LYMPHADENECTOMY STANDARD OF CARE
MESENCHYMAL TUMORS OF THE UTERINE CORPUS
25% ENDOMETRIAL STROMAL SARCOMA
"LOW GRADE" IS THE CURRENT DEFINITION AS "HIGH GRADE" IS NOW REFERRED TO AS. UNDIFFERENTIATED UTERINE SARCOMA
HORMONAL THERAPIES FOUND TO BE EFFECTIVE WITH SOME SUBTYPES
66.6% LEIOMYO-SARCOMA
MOST COMMON IF CARCINOSARCOMA EXCLUDED
HORMONE EXPOSURE
USUALLY POSTOP DIAGNOSIS
MOST COMMONLY PRESENTS AS:
AUB
FLESHY PROTRUDING MASS
ENLARGED UTERUS
D AND C GOLD STANDARD
>90% LINING REPRESENTED
EMB TEST OF CHOICE ~90% REPRESENTED

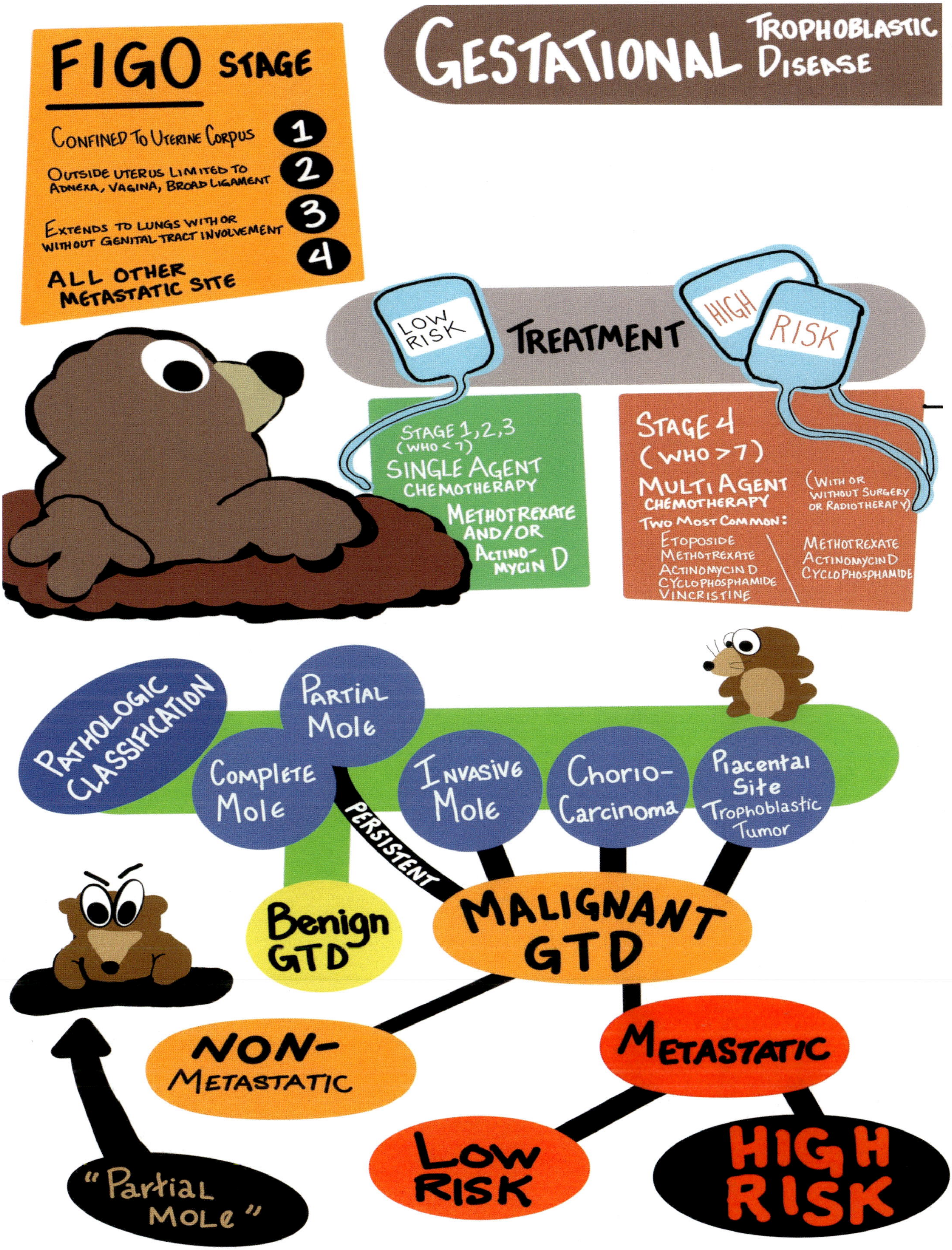
GESTATIONAL TROPHOBLASTIC DISEASE
FIGO STAGE
CONFINED TO UTERINE CORPUS 1
OUTSIDE UTERUS LIMITED TO ADNEXA, VAGINA, BROAD LIGAMENT 2
EXTENDS TO LUNGS WITH OR WITHOUT GENITAL TRACT INVOLVEMENT 3
ALL OTHER METASTATIC SITE 4
TREATMENT
LOW RISK
HIGH RISK
STAGE 1,2,3 (WHO < 7)
SINGLE AGENT CHEMOTHERAPY
METHOTREXATE AND/OR ACTINOMYCIN D
STAGE 4 (WHO > 7)
MULTI AGENT CHEMOTHERAPY
(WITH OR WITHOUT SURGERY OR RADIOTHERAPY)
TWO MOST COMMON:
ETOPOSIDE
METHOTREXATE
ACTINOMYCIN D
CYCLOPHOSPHAMIDE
VINCRISTINE
METHOTREXATE
ACTINOMYCIN D
CYCLOPHOSPHAMIDE
PATHOLOGIC CLASSIFICATION
Partial Mole
Complete Mole
Invasive Mole
Chorio-Carcinoma
Placental Site Trophoblastic Tumor
PERSISTENT
Benign GTD
MALIGNANT GTD
NON-METASTATIC
METASTATIC
Low RISK
HIGH RISK
"Partial MOLE"

Cervical Cancer and PAPS

Here we present the surgical staging of cervical cancer. Cervical cancer is a predictable and usually curable cancer of the female reproductive tract. A women's current chance of being diagnosed with cervical cancer in her lifetime is 0.6%. The current death rate of cancer cases is 2.3 per 100,000 women in a year. The subtypes of these cases are 80% Squamous and 20% are Adenocarcinoma (very rare are Adenosquamous and Clear Cell). The Stages 1A2 and 2A are famous exam questions regarding management. The new addition to the staging is using CT scan for visualizing spread in stage 2 and higher.

Important things to remember on the exam are the C's of Cervical Cancer!

- -CLINICAL staging
- -CISPLATIN for treatment
- -Identifiable CAUSE is CERVICAL HPV
- -CIGARETTES are a high risk factor

TIP:
At Stage 1B the lesion is clinically visible!

"At 1B I can see!"

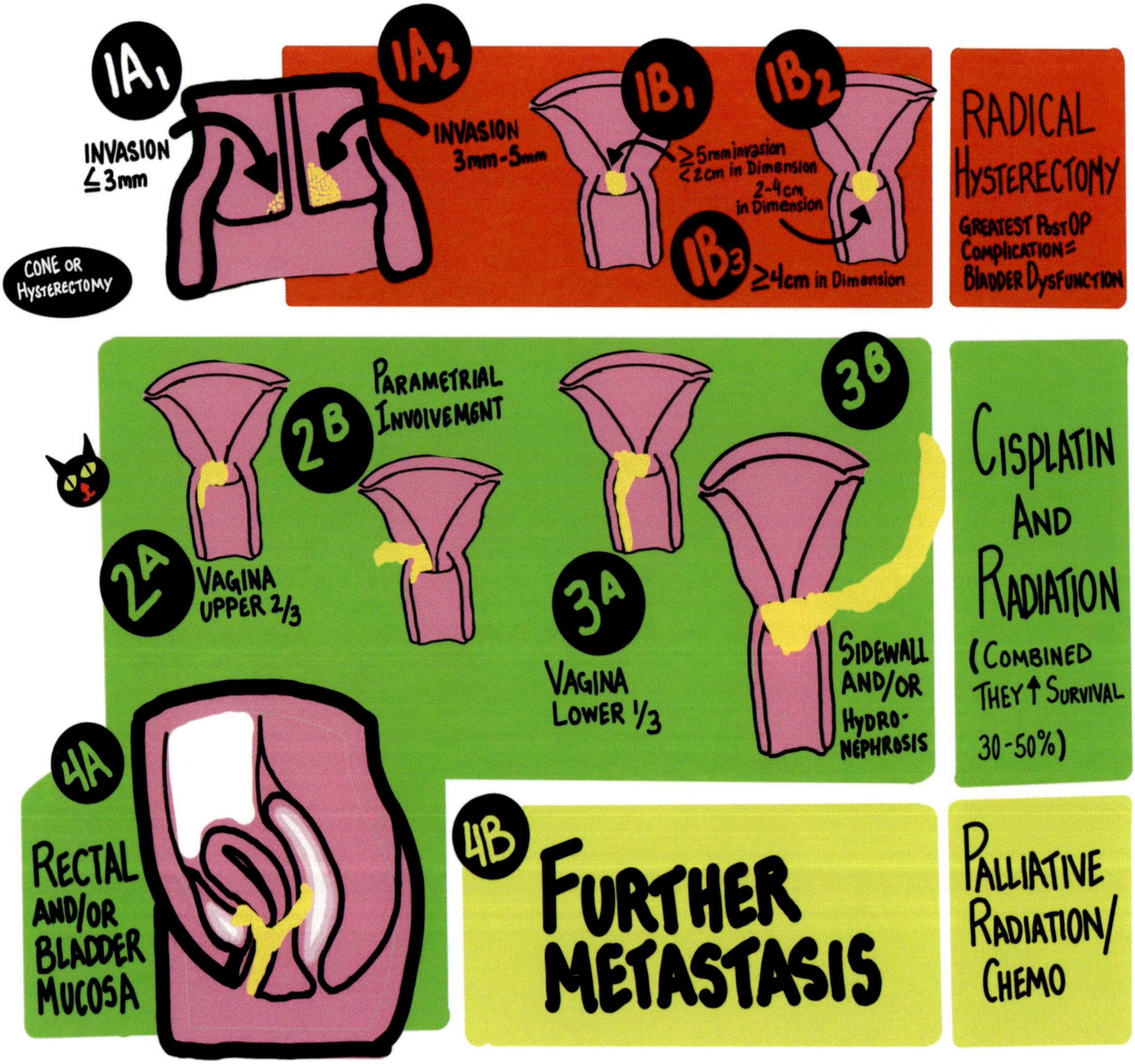

PAPS

SQUAMOUS

CIN 1
- HPV EFFECT
- ASC-US
- LSIL ◄ NEG — P16 IHC STAIN

CIN 2
- HSIL ◄ POS — P16 IHC STAIN
- ASC-H

CIN 3
- CARCINOMA IN-SITU

GLANDULAR

- ATYPICAL GLANDULAR CELLS
- ADENOCARCINOMA
- ADENOCARCINOMA IN SITU
- ENDOMETRIAL CELLS (FEMALE >40 YEARS OLD)

HPV

DS DNA VIRUS

ANOGENITAL
- CONDYLOMA (6, 11)
- DYSPLASIA/CANCER
  - HIGHEST RISK 16, 18
  - (31, 33, 35, 45, 51, 56)

E6 ⊣ P53 (NEEDED FOR APOPTOSIS)

E7 → RETINOBLASTOMA (Rb) PROTEIN → E2F → ↑ CELLULAR PROLIFERATION

INCREASED RISK
- BLACK
- HISPANIC
- ALCOHOL
- HIGHER NUMBER SEX PARTNERS

Squamous

ASC-US

- Relatively common
- 5% paps

CIN 1,2,3...20-30%
CIN 2,3...5-17%
Carcinoma 0.1-0.2%

ASC-US → Repeat Cytology 12 Months
- (−) → 3 year screening
- ASC-US or Greater → Colposcopy

ASC-US → Reflex HPV
- (+) → Colposcopy
- (−) → Repeat CoTest 3 years

ASC-H

Literally CANNOT rule out High Grade Disease!!!

CIN 2,3
40%

ASC-H → Colposcopy! Regardless of HPV (No Reflex)

LSIL

CIN 2
or Greater
12-16%

Similar to behavior to ASC-US HPV +

LSIL → Colposcopy

HSIL

CIN 2
Or Greater
53-66%

Pregnant? Often sent to Gyn-Onc and colpo each T/M

HSIL → Colposcopy / LEEP

Colposcopy:
- (+) → LEEP
- (−) → Colposcopy/Cytology every 6 months for 2 years; 2 negatives can return to routine
- HSIL persists 2 years → LEEP

GLANDULAR

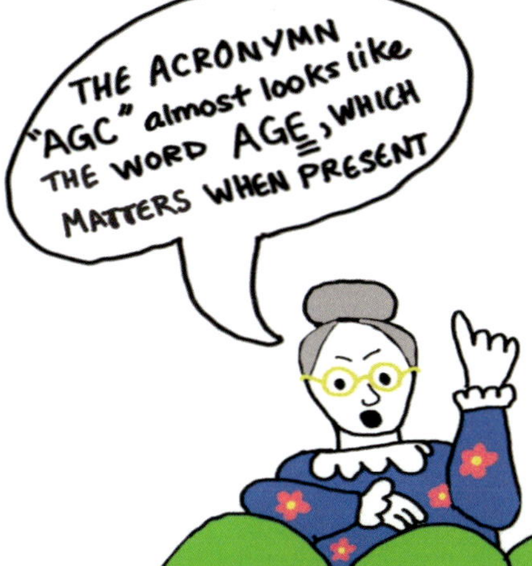
THE ACRONYMN "AGC" almost looks like THE WORD AGE, WHICH MATTERS WHEN PRESENT

AGC in a Premenopausal woman:
More likely to be: HSIL
AGC in a POSTmenopausal woman:
More likely to be:
Adenocarcinoma

AGC

CONCERNS FROM AGC include:

- CIN
- ENDOMETRIAL ADENOCARCINOMA
- CERVICAL ADENOCARCINOMA

AGC

↓

Colposcopy with ECC

With/without EMB:
- menorrhagia
- >35 years old
- <35 years old with:
  - Chronic anovulation
  - Unexplained Vaginal Bleeding

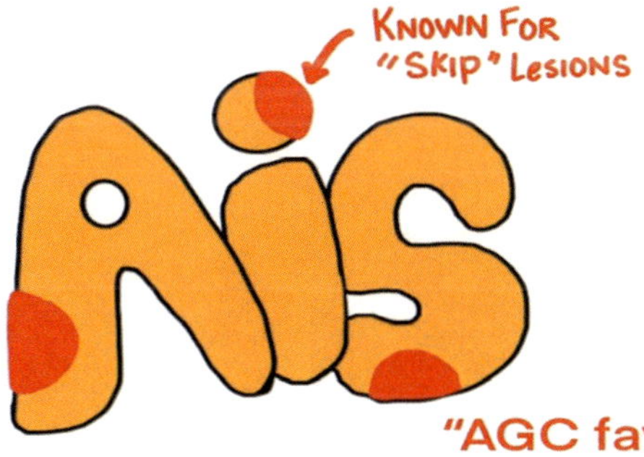
AIS
KNOWN FOR "SKIP" LESIONS

"AGC favors Neoplasia"
Consider GYN-ONC

AIS

→ Colposcopy with ECC with/without EMB (See above)

→ Cold Knife Cone

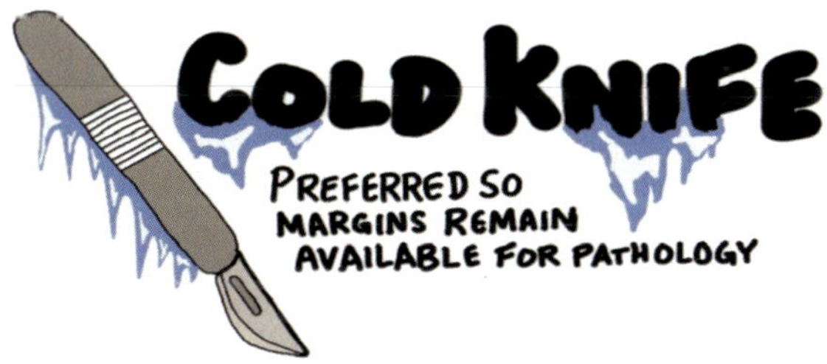
COLD KNIFE
PREFERRED SO MARGINS REMAIN AVAILABLE FOR PATHOLOGY

AGC

- No CIN 2, AIS or Cancer → Co-test 12 and 24 months
- CIN 2 Without glandular Neoplasia → Return to ASCCP Guidelines

HEREDITARY CANCER SYNDROMES

ALL OF THESE ARE AUTOSOMAL DOMINANT

SYNDROME	BREAST	OVARIAN	ENDO-METRIAL	COLON	OTHERS
(HBOC) BRCA 1/2	BRCA1	BRCA2			
LYNCH		MLH1	MSH2	●	GASTRIC URETERAL BILIARY PANCREATIC GLIOBLASTOMA
LI-FRAUMENI	P53				SARCOMA BONE BRAIN ADRENOCORTICAL
COWDEN	Pten		●	●	THYROID BENIGN HAMARATOMAS
PEUTZ JEGHER	STK11	●		● (HAMARTOMAS)	CERVIX PANCREAS GASTRIC

You should know exactly which of the cancer types belong to each syndrome. At least the easy part is that they are ALL AUTOSOMAL DOMINANT, so that's one less thing to remember! Inside the black dots are gene markers that are important to each syndrome in the row (not specific cancers in columns).

REPRODUCTIVE ENDOCRINOLOGY AND INFERTILITY

Cholesterol Synthesis

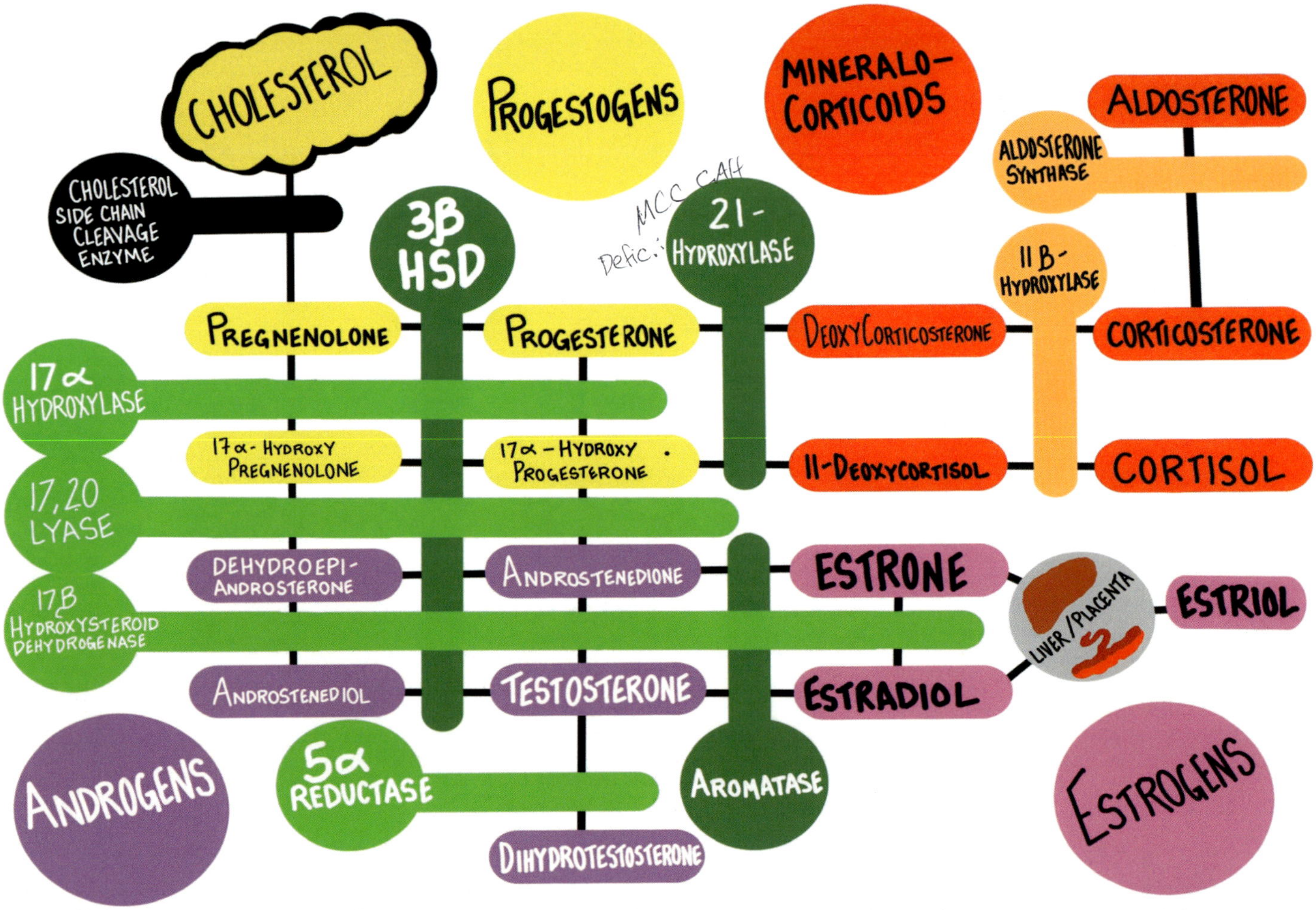

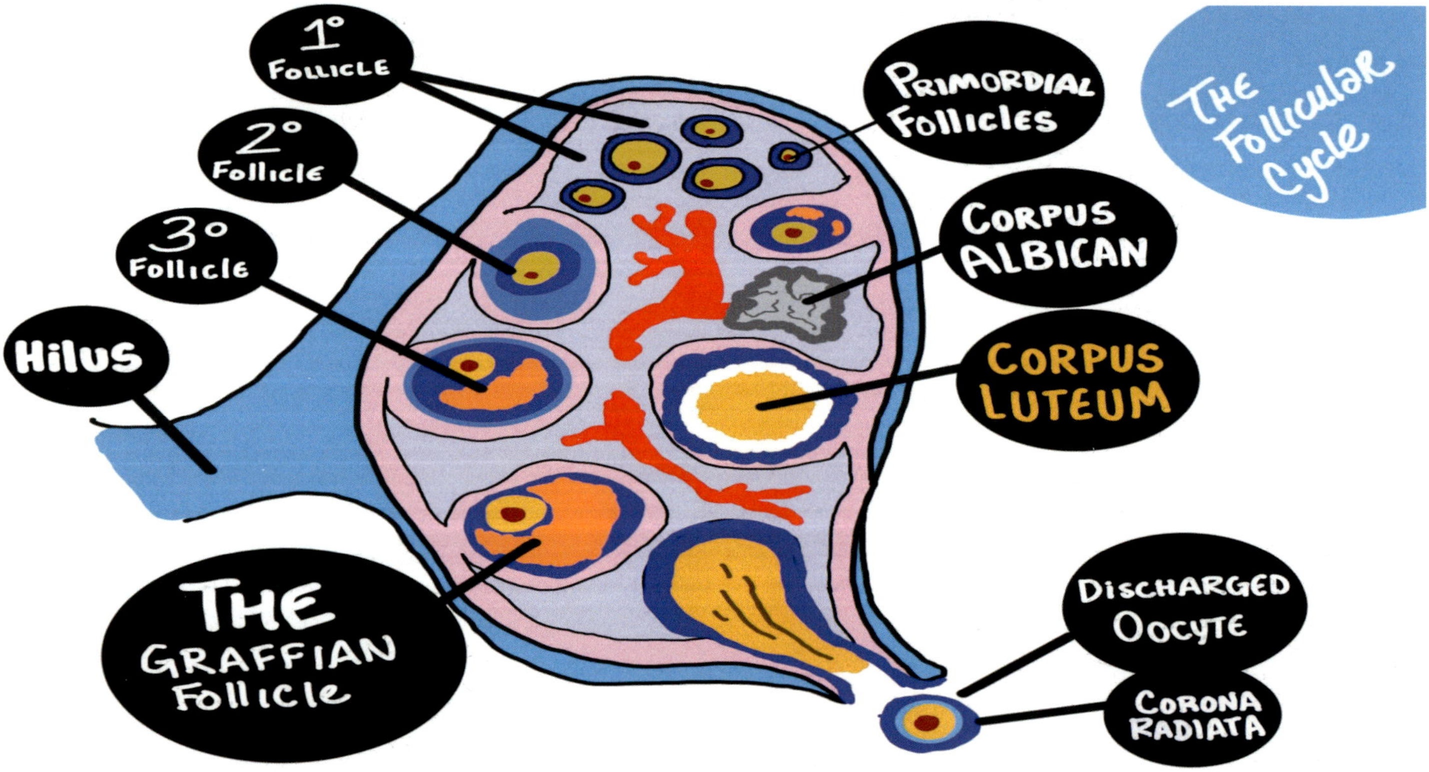

The Menstrual Cycle

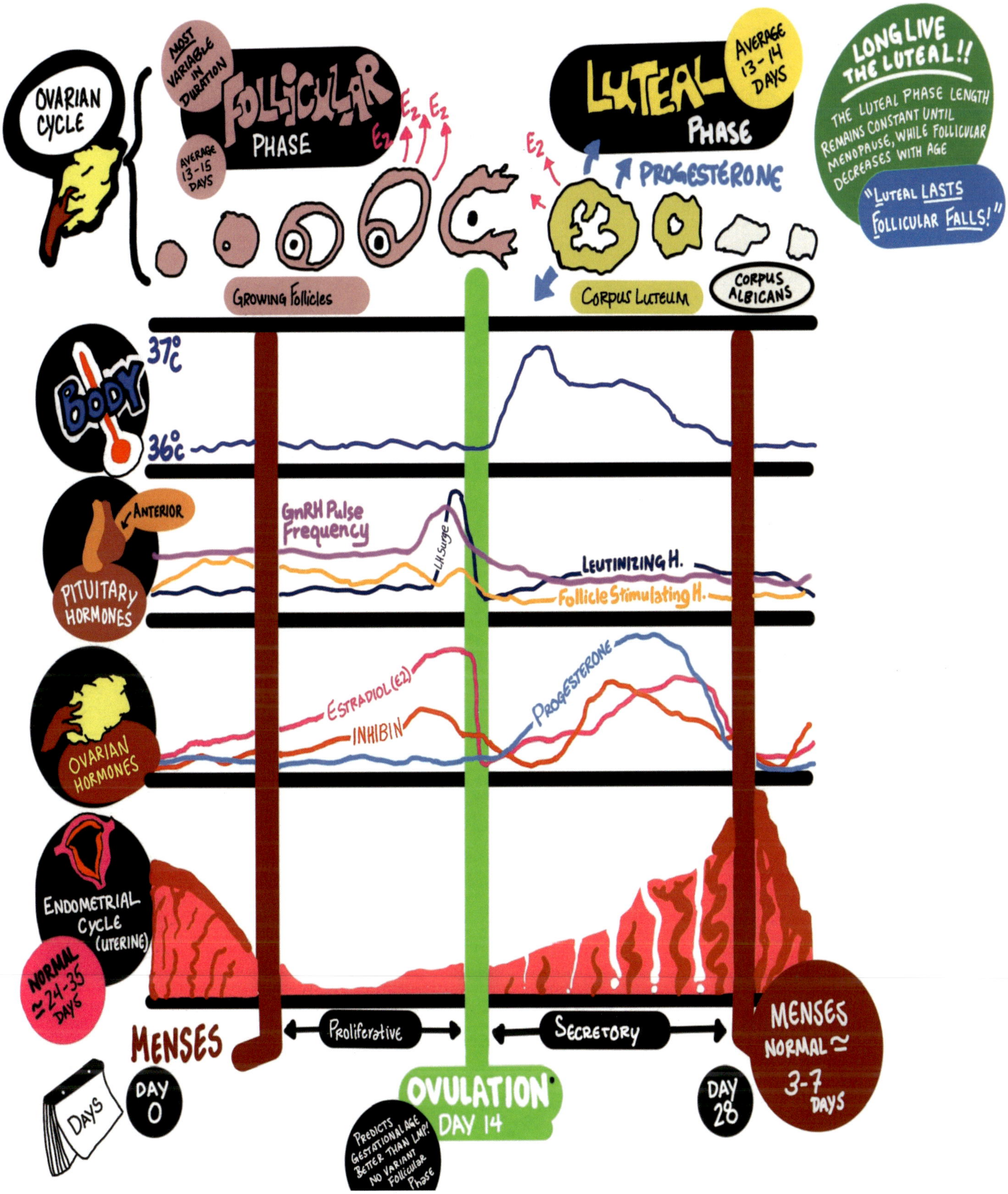

Ovarian Hyperstimulation Syndrome

The processes used to stimulate the ovaries with gonadotrophs for oocyte collection in the infertility process can lead to this syndrome. The releasing of factors such as Vascular Endothelial Growth Factor (VEGF), Interleukin-6 and 8 (IL-6, IL-8), into the blood stream leads to capillary leakage. This subsequently produces tissue edema and hypovolemia. The sequela of these, if not managed and noted immediately, can be life threatening.

Quick recognition and treatment are key to minimizing the risks of this condition.

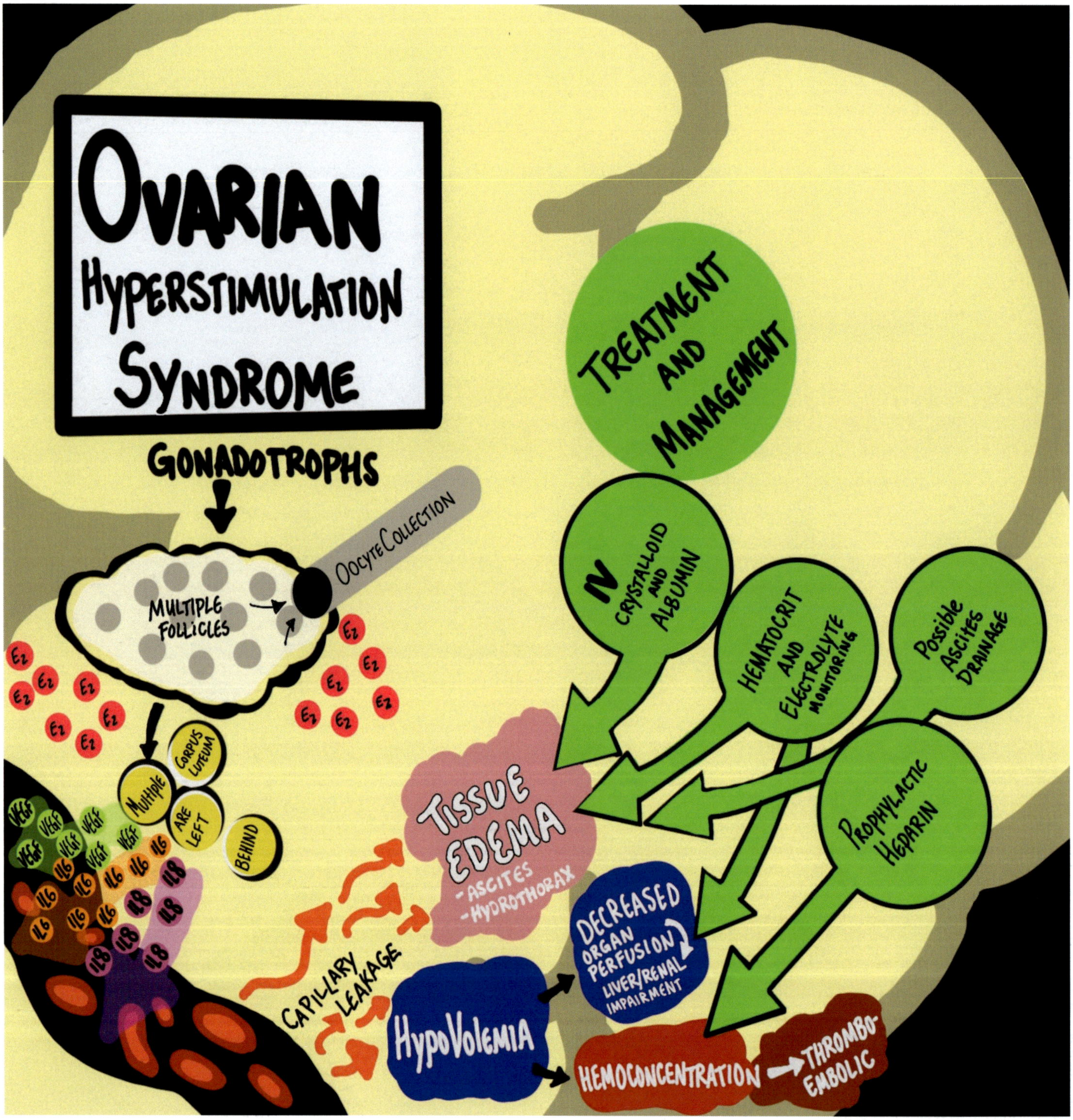

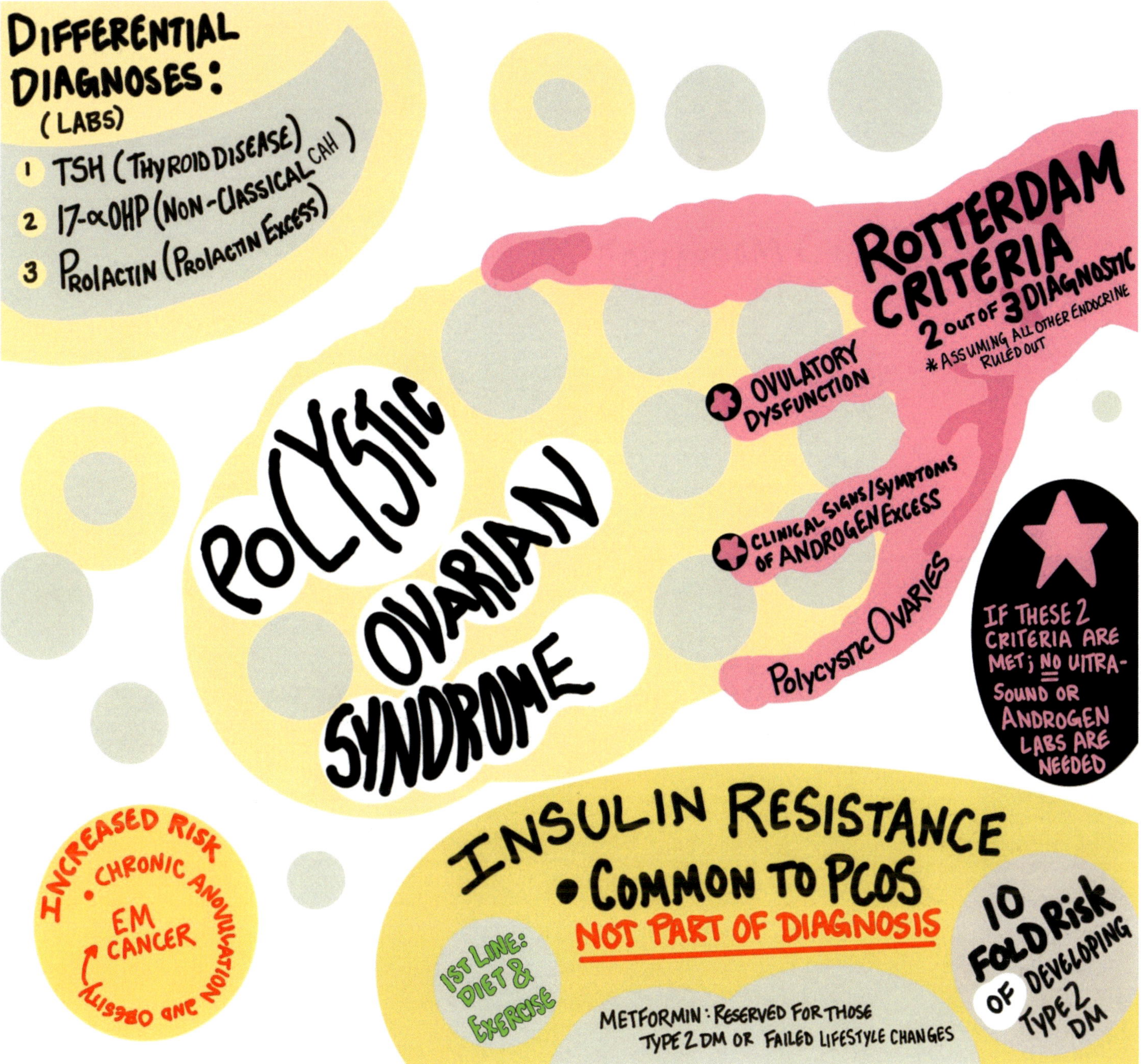

Polycystic Ovarian Syndrome (PCOS)

PCOS is one of the most commonly worked up syndromes in some OB/GYN populations. Understanding this syndrome, the diagnosis and workup are vital to answering questions on your exam. Often, questions focus on the intricacies of diagnosis and sequelae.

The patient that presents with signs/symptoms of ovulatory dysfunction and androgen excess do NOT require further imaging or androgen labs for diagnosis. Also, when diagnosing PCOS you must exclude all other possible endocrine disturbances by using the labs recommended in the upper right corner of the drawing.

Another key point to know is that insulin resistance is COMMON to PCOS. However, it is NOT part of the diagnosis. Also, if Insulin Resistance is diagnosed the FIRST LINE treatment is **Diet and Exercise** NOT medications!

Metabolic Syndrome

You MUST be able to diagnose this syndrome and recognize it in examinations. The key is knowing that 3 out of the 5 are required for a diagnosis. The exam questions usually use numeric values to throw you off or a "like" variable to confuse you. Common "like" variables are LDL, HgbA1c, Neck Circumference, BMI and Cholesterol.

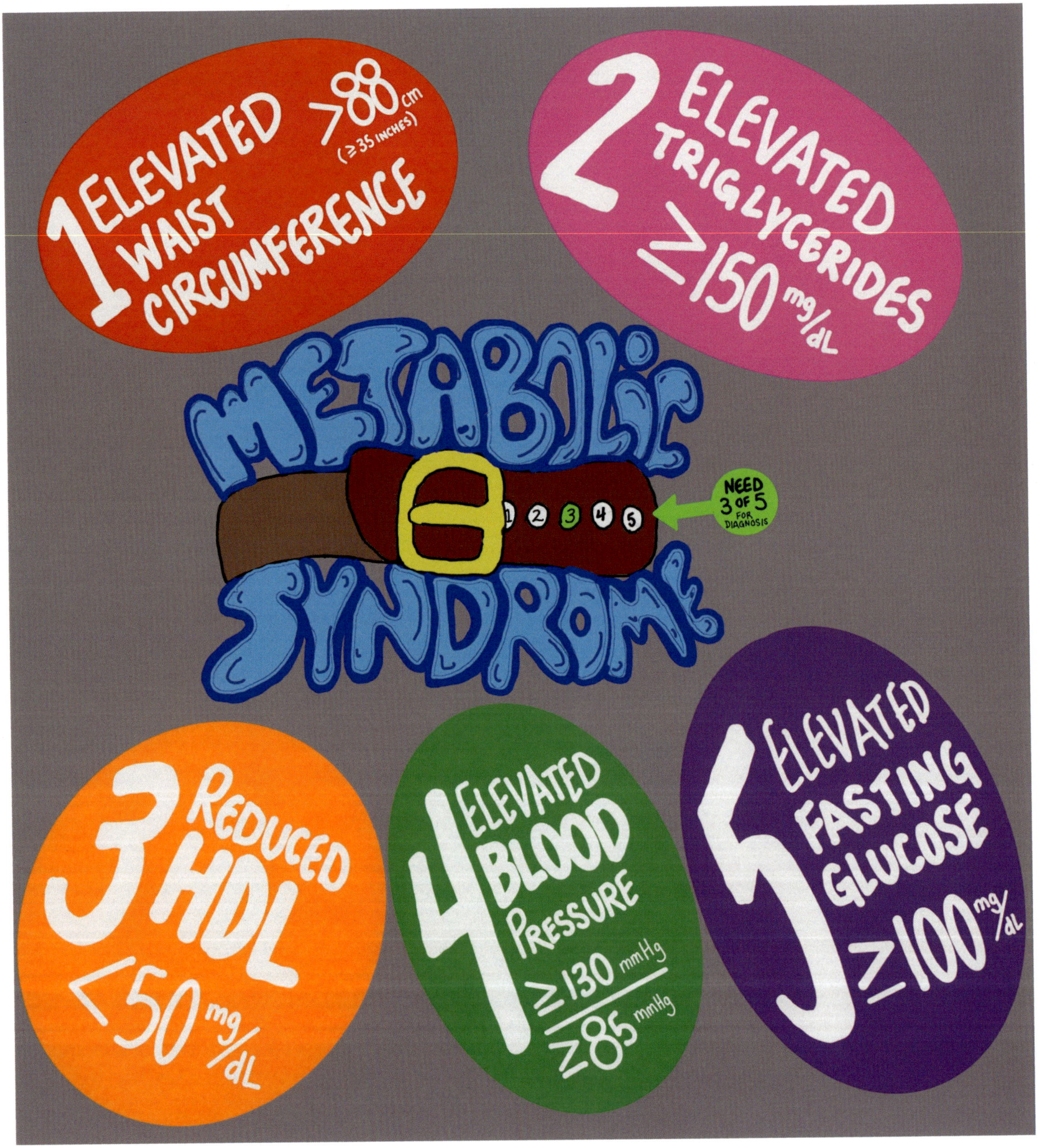

Adrenal Gland

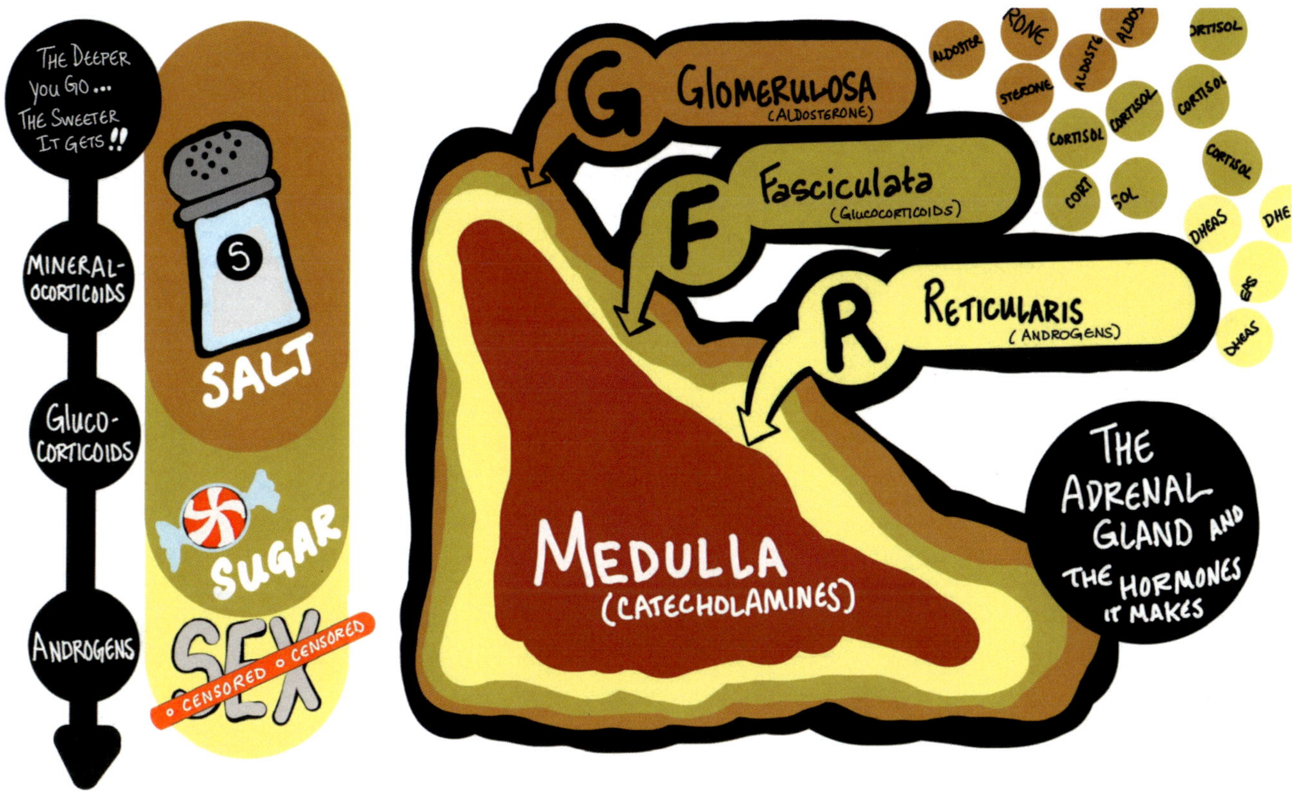

Fetal Adrenal

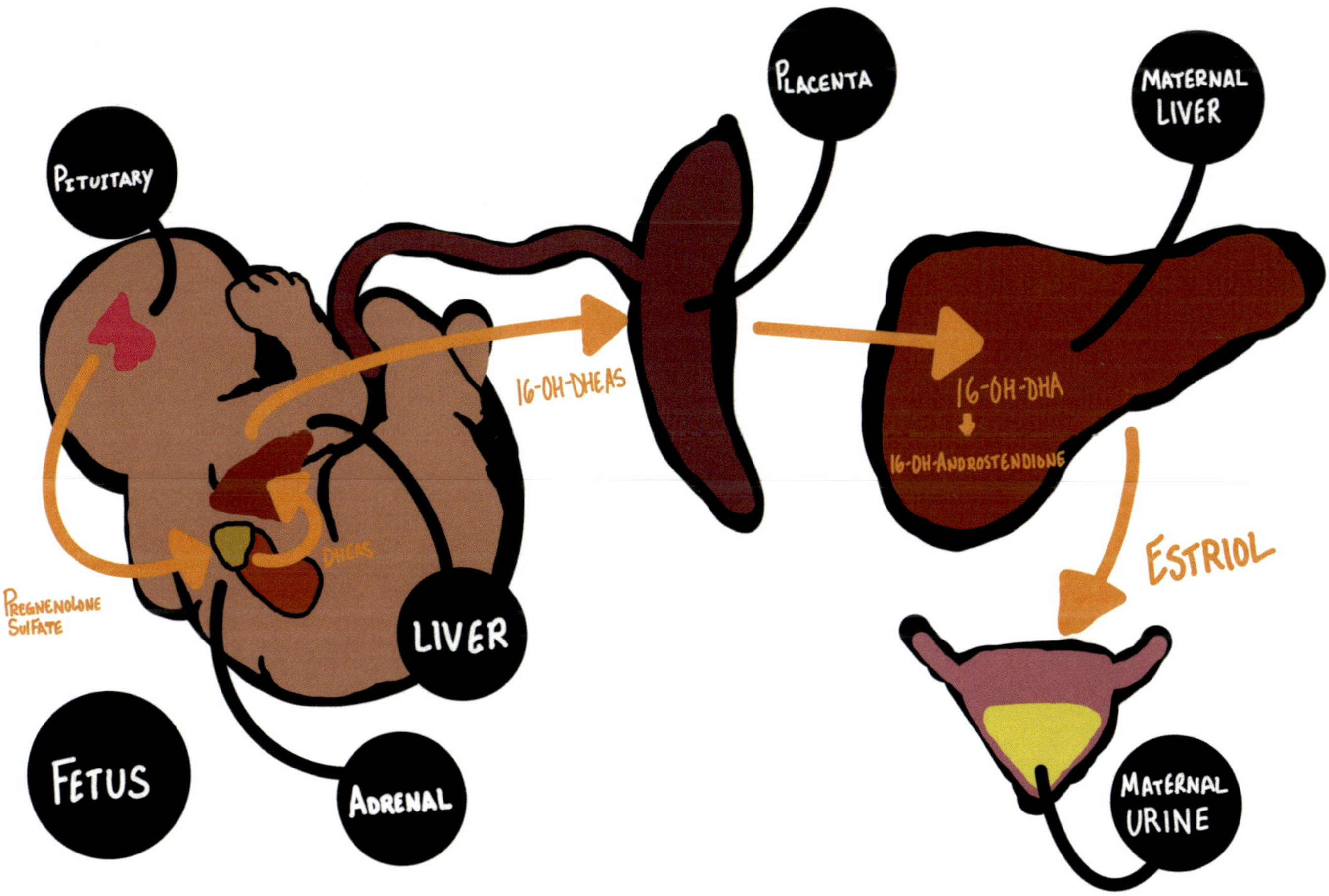

Puberty

Puberty is an important predictor of normal sexual development. If the process is slowed, or accelerated, then differentials should be developed. You must know normal development to be able to spot the abnormal.

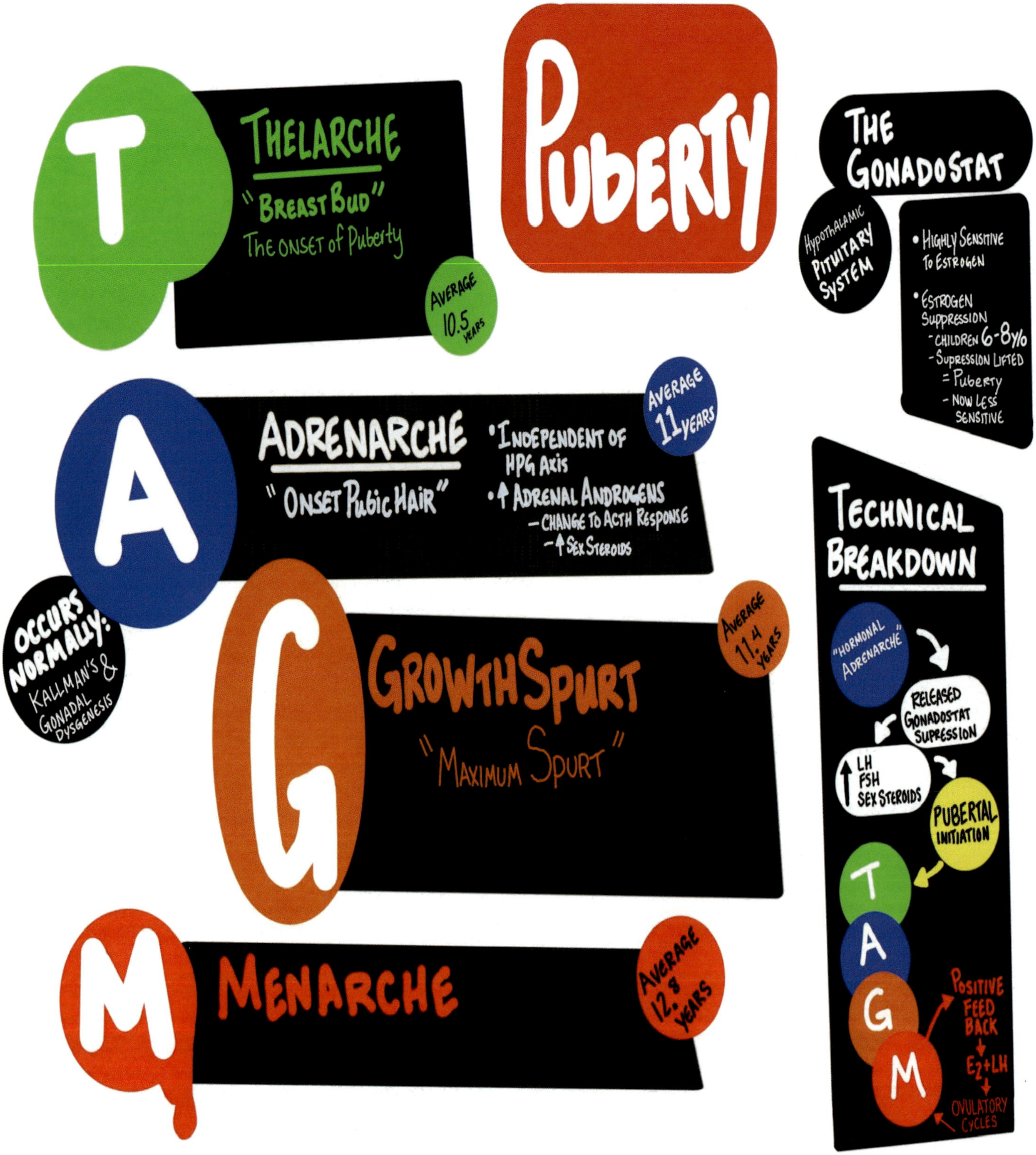
Puberty
T
Thelarche
"Breast Bud"
The onset of Puberty
Average 10.5 years
A
Adrenarche
"Onset Pubic Hair"
• Independent of HPG Axis
• ↑ Adrenal Androgens
– Change to ACTH Response
– ↑ Sex Steroids
Average 11 years
Occurs normally: Kallman's & Gonadal Dysgenesis
G
Growth Spurt
"Maximum Spurt"
Average 11.4 years
M
Menarche
Average 12.8 years
The Gonadostat
Hypothalamic Pituitary System
• Highly sensitive to Estrogen
• Estrogen Suppression
– Children 6-8 y/o
– Supression lifted = Puberty
– Now less sensitive
Technical Breakdown
"Hormonal" Adrenarche
Released Gonadostat Supression
↑ LH FSH Sex Steroids
Pubertal Initiation
T
A
G
M
Positive Feed Back
E2+LH
Ovulatory Cycles

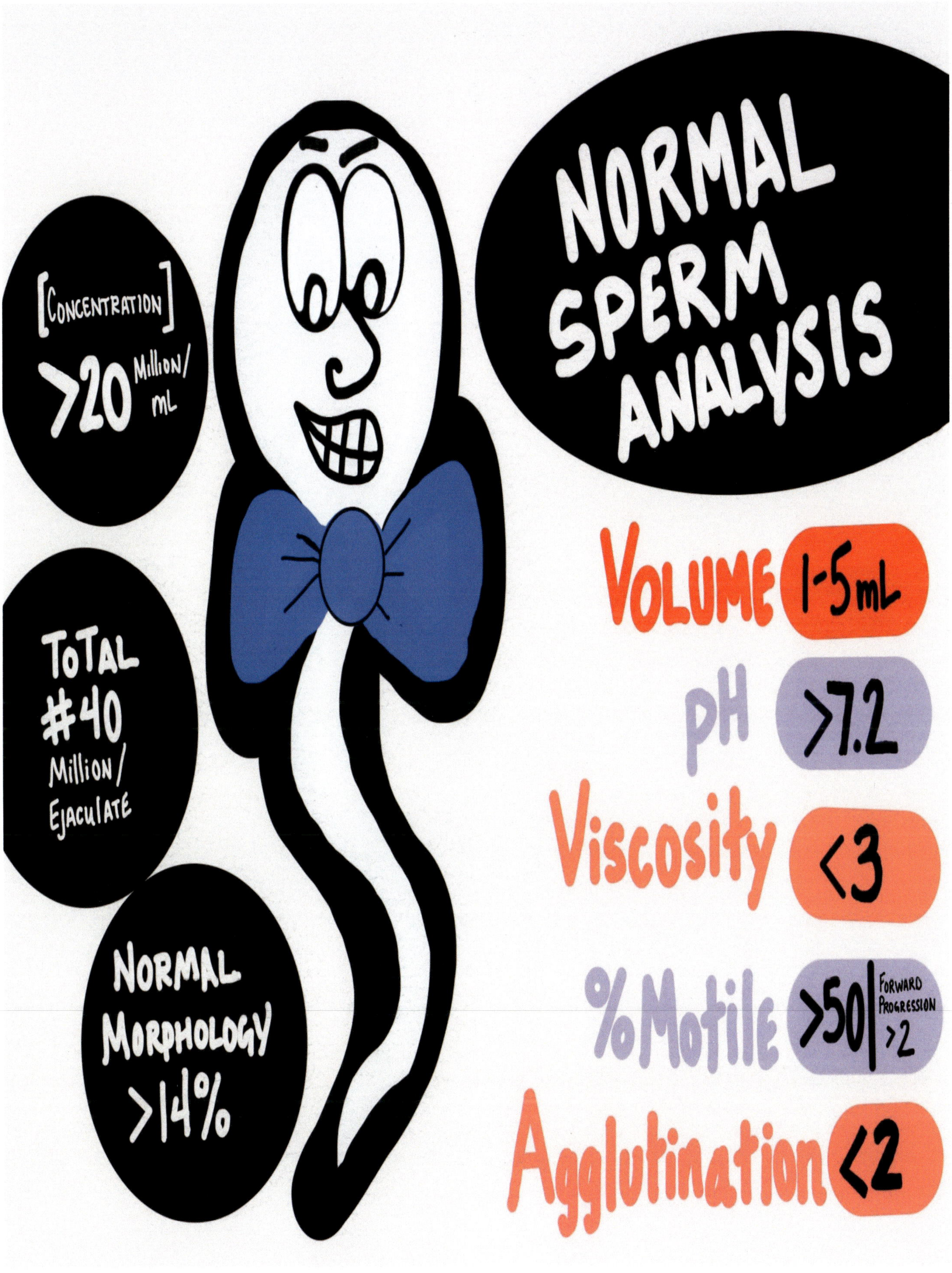
NORMAL SPERM ANALYSIS
[CONCENTRATION]
>20 Million/mL
TOTAL #40 Million/EJACULATE
NORMAL MORPHOLOGY >14%
VOLUME 1-5 mL
pH >7.2
Viscosity <3
% Motile >50 | FORWARD PROGRESSION >2
Agglutination <2

NOTES

BLADDER and INCONTINENCE

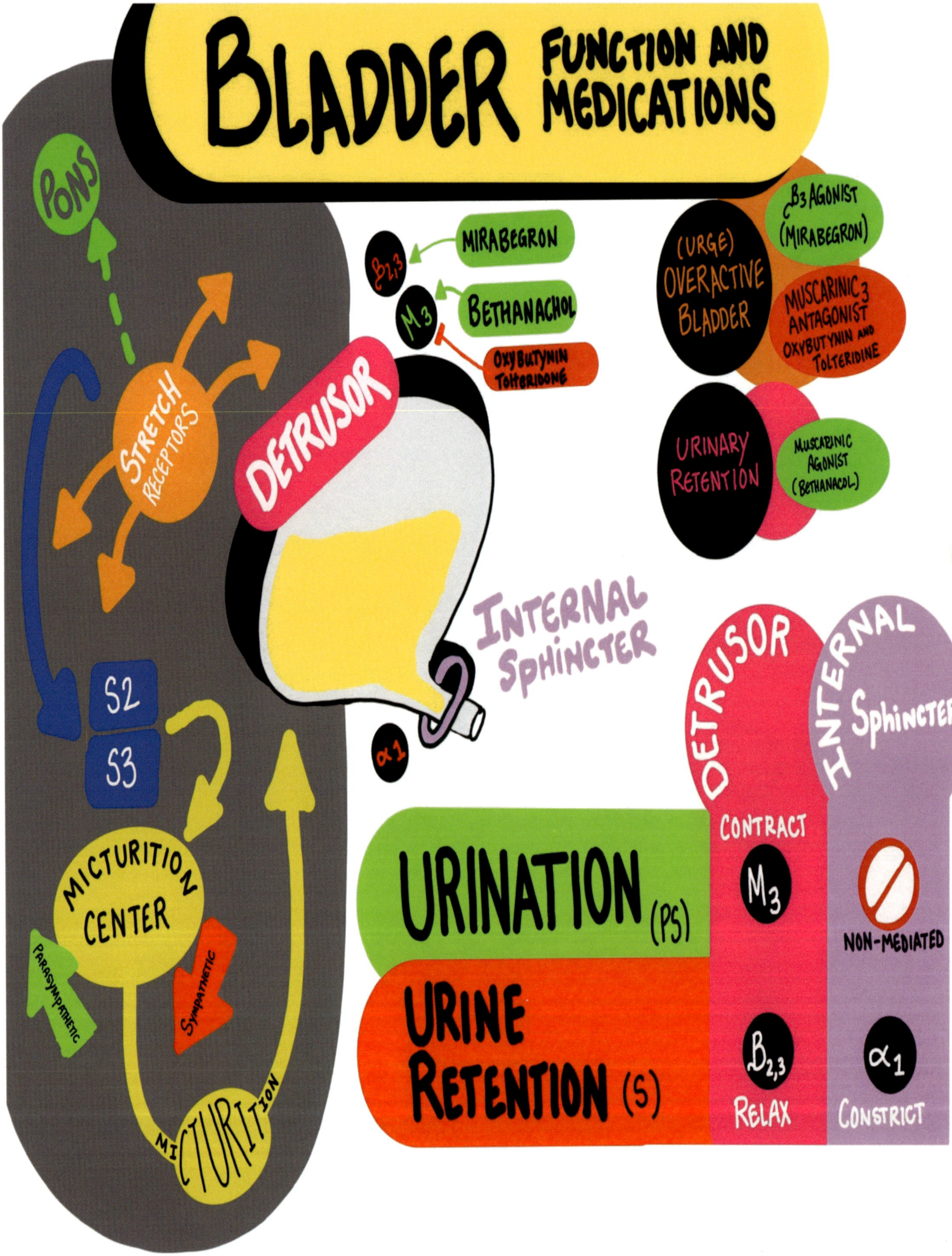
BLADDER FUNCTION AND MEDICATIONS
PONS
STRETCH RECEPTORS
S2
S3
MICTURITION CENTER
Parasympathetic
Sympathetic
MICTURITION
MIRABEGRON
BETHANACHOL
OXYBUTYNIN TOLTERIDONE
$B_{2,3}$
M_3
DETRUSOR
INTERNAL SPHINCTER
$\alpha 1$
(URGE) OVERACTIVE BLADDER
B_3 AGONIST (MIRABEGRON)
MUSCARINIC$_3$ ANTAGONIST OXYBUTYNIN AND TOLTERIDINE
URINARY RETENTION
MUSCARINIC AGONIST (BETHANACOL)
URINATION (PS)
URINE RETENTION (S)
DETRUSOR
INTERNAL Sphincter
CONTRACT
M_3
NON-MEDIATED
$B_{2,3}$
RELAX
α_1
CONSTRICT

Incontinence

The 3 Main Types of Incontinence:

1. Stress Urinary Incontinence
2. Urgency Urinary Incontinence
3. Mixed Urinary Incontinence

Genitourinary Etiology

Filling and Storage Disorders:
- -Urodynamic Stress Disorders
- -Detrusor Overactivity
- -Mixed Types

Fistula

Infectious:
- -Vaginitis
- -UTI

Congenital

Non-genitourinary Etiology

Functional
Environmental
Pharmacologic
Metabolic

Adapted from ACOG PB 155

This topic has become increasingly more popular on the board examinations. Treatments, contraindications to treatments and the adverse effects of surgical interventions have all been stressed.

Many women believe that incontinence is a shameful thing to discuss or something they just have to live with as a natural part of aging.

So, learning the urinary system, and the pathology that affects it, will greatly assist you in your everyday practice and improve the happiness of your patients.

Incontinence risk factors include: Medications, Obesity, Diuretics, Constipation, Diabetes, Smoking, Estrogen Depletion and many others.

OBESITY is an INDEPENDENT RISK FACTOR for incontinence. Per ACOG PB #155 there is a 4.2 FOLD INCREASED RISK of stress urinary incontinence. Weight loss alone in some obese women results in a reduction of incontinence.

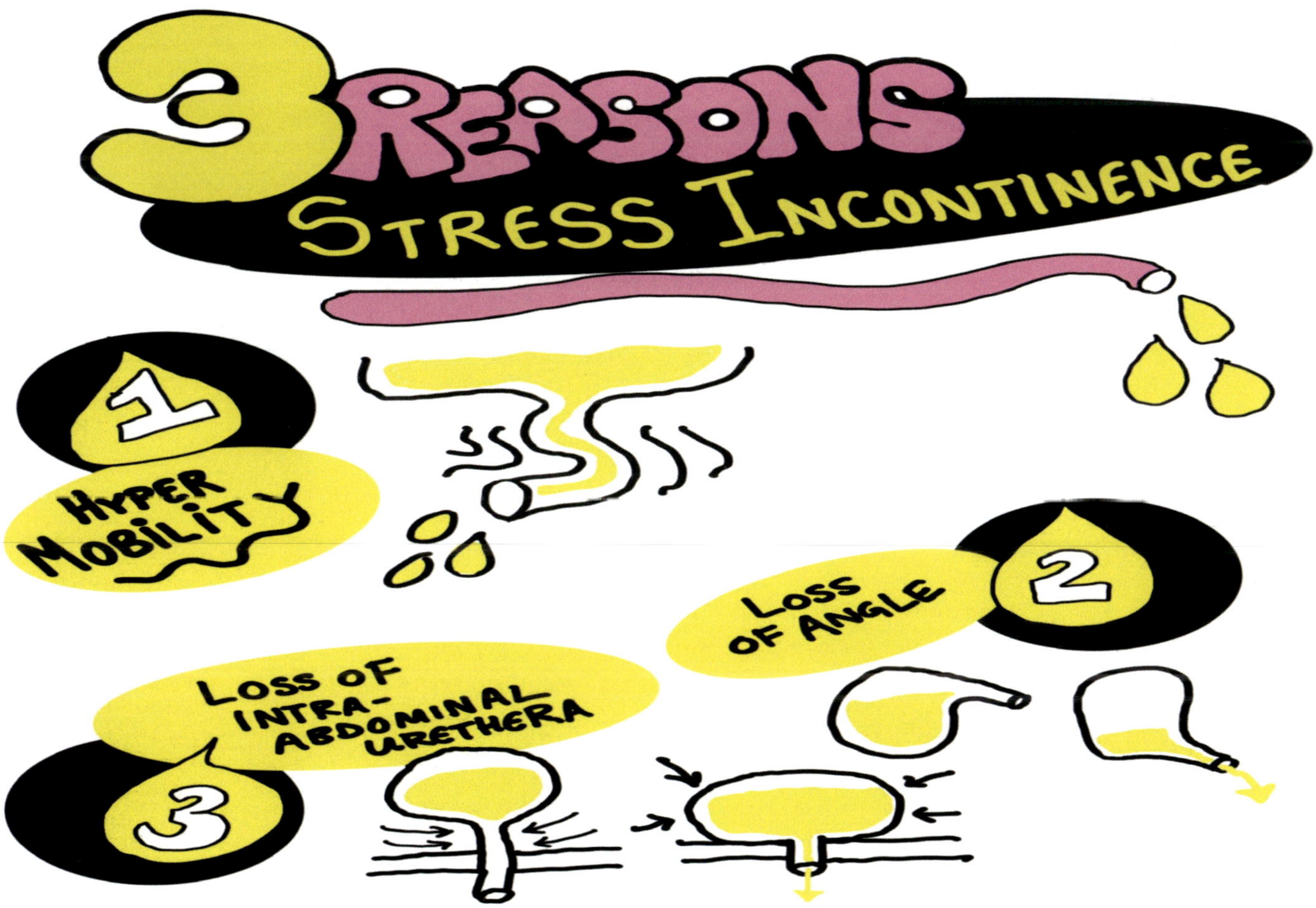
3 REASONS
STRESS INCONTINENCE
1
HYPER MOBILITY
2
LOSS OF ANGLE
3
LOSS OF INTRA-ABDOMINAL URETHERA

Reversible Forms of Incontinence

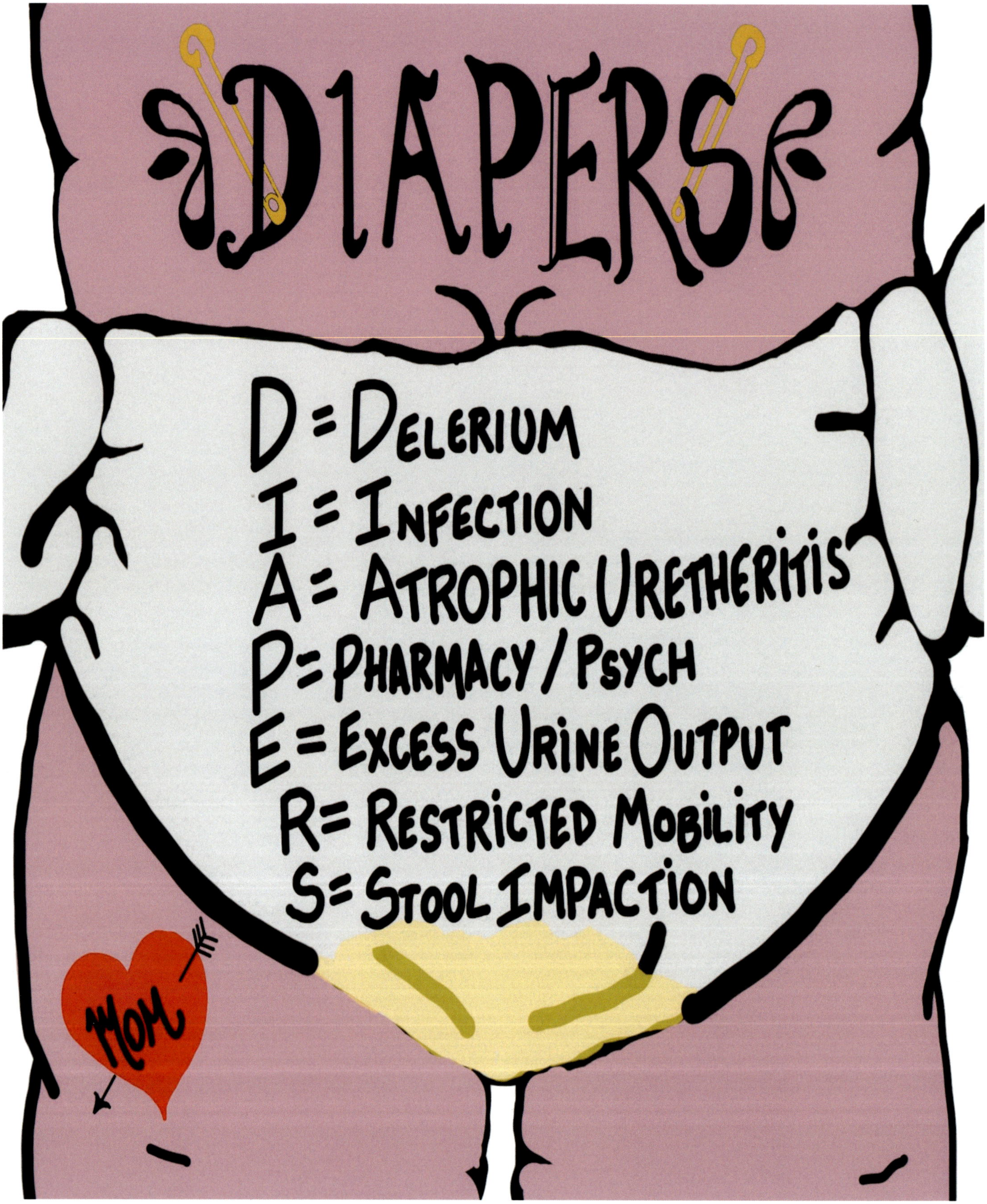

Other Info...

Fruit Salad

This drawing is a culmination of all the things we like to associate with food in our field! They can be helpful facts to remember and the drawing will help you recall these facts! The best use of this drawing is to make yourself familiar with the topics it represents and then quiz yourself on the basket.

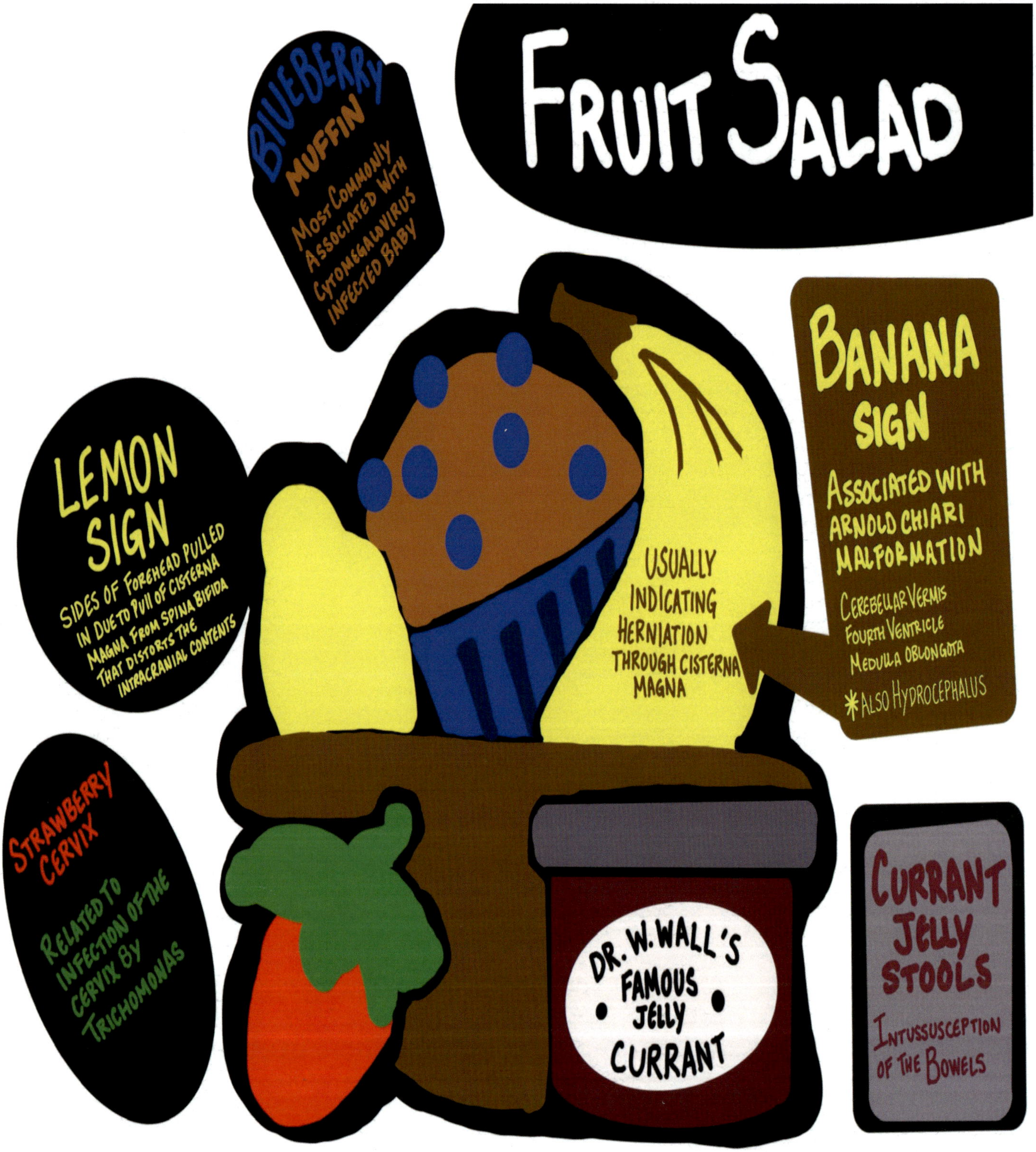

FRUIT SALAD
BLUEBERRY MUFFIN
MOST COMMONLY ASSOCIATED WITH CYTOMEGALOVIRUS INFECTED BABY
LEMON SIGN
SIDES OF FOREHEAD PULLED IN DUE TO PULL OF CISTERNA MAGNA FROM SPINA BIFIDA THAT DISTORTS THE INTRACRANIAL CONTENTS
BANANA SIGN
ASSOCIATED WITH ARNOLD CHIARI MALFORMATION
CEREBELLAR VERMIS
FOURTH VENTRICLE
MEDULLA OBLONGOTA
* ALSO HYDROCEPHALUS
USUALLY INDICATING HERNIATION THROUGH CISTERNA MAGNA
STRAWBERRY CERVIX
RELATED TO INFECTION OF THE CERVIX BY TRICHOMONAS
DR. W. WALL'S FAMOUS JELLY CURRANT
CURRANT JELLY STOOLS
INTUSSUSCEPTION OF THE BOWELS

Professor Research

The professor's lab is to help you remember and to give you some reference for all those biostats questions that always seem to show up on our exams

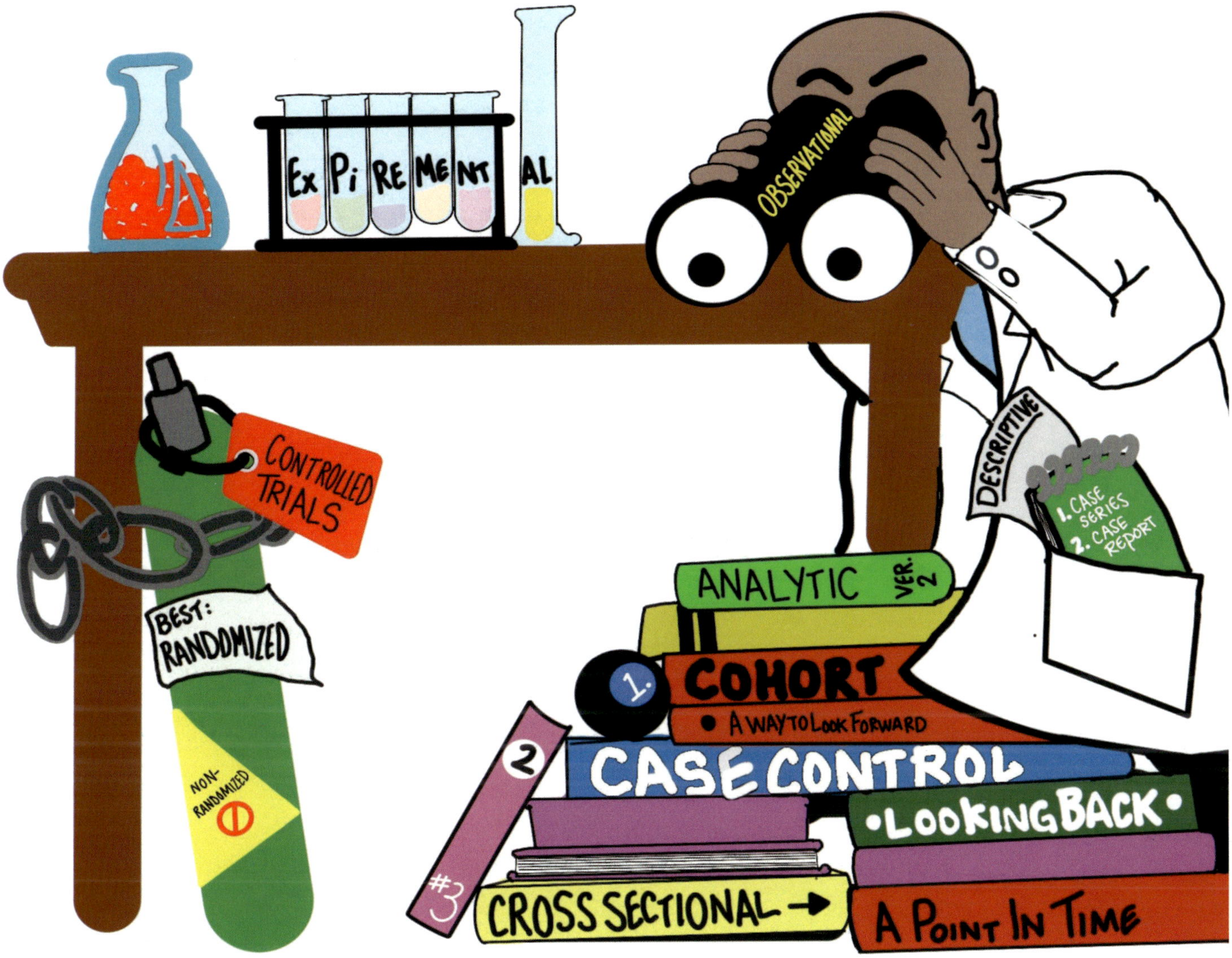

The **LEFT SIDE** of the drawing are

EXPERIMENTAL STUDIES

-Professor's Oxygen Tank shows us
CONTROLLED TRIALS:
-Randomized
-Non-Randomized

Randomized Trials are the Gold Standard

The **RIGHT SIDE** of the drawing are

OBSERVATIONAL STUDIES

-Professor's Coat Pocket holds the
DESCRIPTIVE STUDIES:
-Case Series
-Case Report

-Professor's Book Pile shows you the
ANALYTIC STUDIES:
-Cohort (forward looking Study)
-Case Control (backward looking Study)
-Cross Sectional (point in time study)

INDEX

